THE GOOD
THE BAD AND THE
HEALTHY

NR

SUNNA VAN KAMPEN

Founder of TONIC HEALTH

THE GOOD THE BAD AND THE HEALTHY

How to make smarter daily choices, from what's in your fridge to what's in your bathroom cabinet

NR

Disclaimer

This book is for informational purposes only. It is not intended to serve as a substitute for professional medical advice – it's meant to inform and empower, not to diagnose, cure, prevent, or treat any condition or disease. It doesn't account for your unique medical history or circumstances, so it's essential to check with your care team and a qualified provider before making any changes to how you eat or how you manage your health. The author and publisher expressly disclaim responsibility for any adverse effects that may result from the use or application of the information it contains.

Published in 2026 by New River Books
Unit 105, Leroy House, 436 Essex Road, London N1 3QP
www.newriverbooks.co.uk

10 9 8 7 6 5 4 3 2

Copyright © Sunna van Kampen

A CIP catalogue record for this book is available from the British Library.

ISBN: 978-1-915780-67-6

Printed and Bound in the UK using 100% Renewable Electricity at CPI Group (UK) Ltd, Croydon, CR0 4YY.

Cover design: Smith & Gilmour
Editorial Consultant: Louise Atkinson

This FSC© label means that materials used for the product have been responsibly sourced.

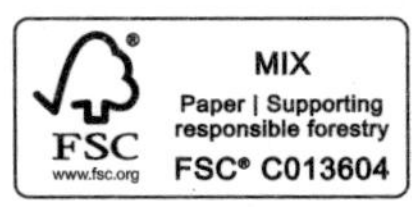

Where images or quotes have been used in this text, every effort has been made to contact copyright holders and abide by 'fair use' guidelines. If you are a copyright holder and wish to get in touch, please email info@newriverbooks.co.uk

CONTENTS

INTRODUCTION

The weekly supermarket shop is one of those rituals that quietly underpins all of our lives. It is at once routine and essential: bread and milk, the rows of fresh fruit and vegetables, the shelves stacked with temptations. The choices made here ripple far beyond the checkout – they form the foundation of our families' health and long-term wellbeing.

For many of us, the trip can feel like a chore. By the time I hit the supermarket, my head is full of competing demands – work deadlines, the children, what on earth to cook for supper, and whether or not we've run out of bin bags.

But nowadays, I try to pause and see this time differently. The supermarket is not just a place of stress and expenditure. It is a kind of ground zero: where habits are formed, where the week ahead is shaped, where the decision between wholesome and harmful is made in the space of a few moments. For me, it has also become a time of connection. Safely strapped in the trolley seat so he can't dart away, my son often joins me, and we negotiate the aisles together. I remind myself that every choice I make is a lesson he is absorbing. If I can focus on calm, deliberate decisions, choosing more of the good and less of the bad without breaking the bank, then I'm giving my kids a small gift that goes beyond the shopping bag.

The weekly shop certainly matters more than we think. It is not simply about filling cupboards. It is where you take the first steps to invest in your health.

But it wasn't always this way for me. Everyone's health journey is different, but all of us start out rejecting broccoli and wanting to eat all the sweets and chocolate we can find, don't we? I was certainly no different. As a teenager I believed I was invincible – McDonalds was my idea of food heaven.

For many people, myself included, there will be something or someone that stops us in our tracks and makes us think differently about food and health. Perhaps it's when you become a parent, or you get struck by a health scare, or maybe when you turn a milestone age.

That's when you might wake up to the realisation that what you put into your body is going to have a very big effect on your life.

The Lemsip years

My first jolt happened at 24. I was living the city life and burning the candle at both ends. I thought I was healthy. I played lots of sport and ate lots of protein, but I noticed I was coming down with four or five colds each winter. When friends and work colleagues started to ask, 'Didn't you have a cold last month?' I knew I had to do something. I spoke to my GP, who referred me to a nutritionist. Blood tests revealed that, even though I thought I was eating healthily, there simply wasn't enough nutritional goodness in my diet. In fact, there were significant nutrient deficiencies that needed to be corrected if I wanted to fuel my immune system and allow it to function properly.

This fascinated me and I went down a massive research rabbit hole, reading all the scientific studies I could lay my hands on to understand why my diet was deficient and how I could correct that. I discovered that, according to science, supporting my immune system required *optimal* levels of nutrition. So I started popping vitamins, but when I scanned the labels, it occurred to me that every supplement was basing its formulation on Nutrient Reference Value (NRV) or Recommended Daily Allowance (RDA), which is the *minimum* amounts of each nutrient you need to avoid deficiency diseases – not the amounts we really need for optimal health.

Healing my girl

Around the same time, my girlfriend (now wife) Anya Garnis was diagnosed with a chronic autoimmune condition called ulcerative colitis. The thought of taking steroids for the rest of her life and never being comfortable eating out again was frankly too life-changing for us to accept.

I dug deeper into health research and nutrition and it became my obsession. This was around 2016, long before gut health was a trendy topic, so the information wasn't widely available.

Anya and I both scoured health books and scientific papers looking for any glimmer of hope that could mean she could live and eat normally, without relying on a cocktail of drugs. We saw numerous specialists, including one in Los Angeles, who charged $2,000 for a consultation just to tell Anya that she should be eating plain foods like bread and potatoes, dismissing my argument that these foods would be low in nutrients.

We ended up taking things into our own hands with an experimental approach, adjusting our meals and paying close attention to how Anya's body responded. For example, we came up with a morning smoothie that combined raw honey, aloe vera, water kefir (for probiotics) and lime juice (for taste) alongside L-glutamine and colostrum supplementation. My mum has always been a big believer in natural remedies, so I also knew from her repertoire that honey has often been used in traditional wound healing (it turns out the science now exists for this too).[1]

Amazingly, Anya's condition went into remission and has stayed there ever since. This made it abundantly clear to me that, if you feed your body with the right fuel and nutrients, it has an incredible power to heal itself. It is just that we live in a food environment that hinders health issues rather than helps them – and a medical environment that believes pharmaceutical drugs provide the best answer.

With Anya now healthy, I threw all my research and passion for optimal health into launching my own vitamin brand, Tonic Health, with a promise of optimal nutrition providing a feast of vitamins, minerals, nutrients and plant extracts with no added sugar, sweeteners, or fillers. We must be doing something right because Tonic has really taken off – it has been the fastest growing vitamin brand in the UK for the last two years.

Let's hear it for my dad

The final piece of the puzzle in my own health journey was prompted by my dad, Mouni van Kampen. It was Dad who, without realising it, helped me understand the psychology behind behaviour change.

He was a pretty typical dad – he kept fit playing football right up until his 60s – but as soon as he stopped, his weight crept up and the odd glass of wine on the weekend stretched to weekdays and then became a daily evening ritual, always accompanied by a bag of crisps. I knew this was unhealthy and I begged my dad to change, but he simply wouldn't.

No matter how many scientific studies I dangled under his nose about oily, salty, highly processed snacks, nothing seemed to cut through. It was only when I stumbled on a brand of air-baked cheese – crunchy, delicious little bites made from 100% cheese with no additives – that I managed to make inroads. I bought Dad a subscription box and suggested he swap these for his regular crisps, and that was it!

It turned out my dad needed the glass of wine and something crunchy as a 'treat' at the end of a hard day. It was his much-loved moment of relaxation, and who was I to deny him that pleasure?

The key to unlocking real health change in him was to embrace the lifestyle habits that brought him joy but provide a *slightly* healthier alternative.

That lesson taught me to understand and appreciate

the psychology of change. It made me realise that small, sustainable lifestyle tweaks can be easy for almost anyone, if they're done without too much restriction and plenty of enjoyment.

The next step came when we started posting little health tips on Tonic's social channels. I really enjoyed finding health swaps that were simple, doable, and accessible for everyone, and that's when things really accelerated. My mini videos went viral – within just a few days some were getting 250k views.

It was clear that the easily actionable health swaps idea resonated, eventually growing into the idea for this book. Thousands of videos later, we are still going into the supermarket each week trying to find ways for you to be healthier. This includes everything from swapping your Malbec for Pinot Noir (cutting 30-50% sugar per glass), to choosing the supermarket own-label cream cheese over the leading branded one (saving you money and cutting out the added gums).

This year, I also started a podcast series called The Unprocessed Truth, where I talk to people from all walks of life about their health journeys. We've interviewed Olympians about how they've reached their sporting heights, and heard from Love Islanders about the perks and pitfalls of getting that Love Island body. We also try and uncover the truth about complicated subjects like microplastics and cholesterol.

The people who really responded to my podcast and posts on TikTok and Instagram kept telling me they wanted to be a little bit healthier, but they didn't have time to read those studies and plough through the books and articles. So, I decided to do the research for them and come up with some simple swaps.

You can follow as many or as few of them as you like, but the more tiny changes you make, the better your health will be!

I'm a dad too

I think it helps that I understand the sort of time and financial pressures so many of my followers share. As a dad of two little ones, aged one and three, I know the struggle. You want to feed them real, nourishing food, but life gets in the way. You're tired, they're picky, and sometimes the easiest thing is to give in. Everywhere you turn, the quick options are the unhealthy ones. Feeding kids well isn't just about food, it's about time, energy and emotion. Some days you win, some days you don't, and that's ok. I find with the one-year-old, I'm still in control. He eats home-cooked food and he gets what he's given. With the three-year-old, this is now the challenge. We get tantrums and stubborn opinions at every meal.

We try to make dinner a real family affair – it's one of the few times in the day we can all sit together. Most evenings, my wife and I trade off cooking duty, or we cook together if the kids give us the space. During the week we aim to keep our dinners simple, healthy, and satisfying. This isn't about fancy or complicated recipes; it's about getting nutritious food on the table without too much fuss or time committed. A typical weeknight dinner might be something like a baked salmon fillet with roasted vegetables, or homemade burgers, salad and pickles. In the winter, I love doing a one-pot slow-cooked lamb stew loaded with carrots, potatoes, and any veg I have in the fridge. Another weekday staple is a sheet-pan meal, where you put chicken thighs, onions, peppers and sweet potatoes (or any other veg for that matter) all tossed on a tray with some olive oil and herbs, then roasted in the oven. It's minimal prep, minimal clean-up and plenty of leftovers for the next day. An easy, healthy meal that takes 5-10 minutes and is made from 100% wholefoods. The idea is to incorporate a variety of vegetables and a source of protein (meat, fish, eggs, or legumes) and that is the basis for our meal. Meat and vegetables. Nothing more, nothing less. We just aim for real, unprocessed foods most of the time and our kids eat the same. For the baby, we'll just whizz up the unseasoned meat and veg, and for the toddler, we might mash the potatoes to increase the chance of him eating them – but broadly we cook one meal for the whole family. Now one thing is clear: you won't win the healthy food battle every night. Sometimes my toddler refuses to eat our food and I confess we don't always have the strength to fight him on it. One off-dinner isn't going to change anything. It's about your consistent actions and the majority of food your kids consume over the many years they're going to spend in your home that make the difference. Anya and I work hard to bring up our two very young children to be as healthy as possible, but we have real lives too! We don't count calories, don't like to limit ourselves on social occasions, or the weekend for that matter, we love dessert and we eat chocolate every day.

Once dinner's done, we involve everyone in that all-important milk-and-choc time. This is our little treat at the end of a long day and another family moment that everyone looks forward to – enjoyed in the living room or outside if the weather allows. It's simply half a glass of local, grass-fed, unhomogenised milk, and two to three pieces of dark chocolate, 85% or 90%. Even our three-year-old loves dark chocolate and looks forward to it every day. It's all about taste-bud training.

It starts with the shopping

For this book, I've chosen to focus on the supermarket because it's somewhere most of us end up each week, making decisions about what to buy and what not to buy. Those decisions provide a unique window onto how we live: they reveal our routines, our cravings, our comforts (like my dad's link between relaxing and a crunchy snack).

And this is where the first changes can be made. The supermarket is where you can choose to push the health of you and your family one notch higher in the priority list. Just by making a few small swaps each time you shop, you can start to make a big and long-lasting health difference.

It's not just about food – those tiny decisions to be a little better and a little healthier extend to what we pick up in other supermarket aisles too: the personal care, cleaning and cooking products too.

My aim is to show you an easier path, a doable middle ground that's not perfect, but it's better than the path you are probably taking. There's no need for draconian choices and a complete life change, but just walk with me around the supermarket and I'll show you simple steps to put you in the right direction.

The low-down on UPFs

If you've watched any of my social media videos, you'll know that I'm pretty passionate about trying to reduce the chemical load we place on our bodies. When I'm suggesting simple swaps to make your shopping basket just a little bit more healthy, I'll be scrutinising the labels on food, cleaning and personal care products to find those with the fewest possible additives, preservatives and potentially harmful compounds.

My message is all about moderation. I'm not going to suggest you stop shopping in the supermarket (where you have so much variety and choice and, often, quite a few bargains) and switch to an eye-wateringly expensive organic wholefoods store all the time. But in the following chapters I can – and will – point out the good stuff (all natural and additive-free), the bad stuff (doused in chemicals), and the thousands of wonderfully healthy options in between.

Because at the end of the day, the occasional pack of cheesy Wotsits won't kill you, and unless you suffer from extreme sensitivities, you're not going to be irreversibly harmed by a supermarket-brand body lotion or sunscreen. But I stand firm in my belief that if you can minimise your chemical exposure – even just reduce it a little bit, week by week – you and your family will be MUCH healthier in the long run.

We might not be able to control the potentially toxic chemicals in the water, or in the air we breathe – but, with my help, you should be able to walk out of the super-market with a slightly reduced chemical load in your shopping bags every time you shop.

What's the problem with ultra-processed food?

I'm certainly not the first person to highlight the potential dangers of eating too many ultra-processed foods (UPFs), and I'm confident I won't be the last. But to make sense of all the healthy food and product swaps I will be suggesting in this book, I need to explain why we all need to seriously cut back on UPFs in our diet.

In the UK, we are among the world's top consumers of UPFs – only behind the US, with 57% of our diets now ultra-processed. Yes, you read that right: over half the calories that Brits consume are from UPFs. That's the pastries, packaged breads, ready meals, crisps, cereals, sweets, fizzy drinks and so on, that form the bulk of many people's breakfasts, lunches and snacks. And it gets worse. Researchers found that children get an even larger share of UPFs.[2] From the ages of two to five, UPFs account for 61% of calories consumed by UK children – a higher proportion than their peers in the US and Australia – making UK kids the world leaders in UPF consumption.

Although our food environment has shifted dramatically in recent decades, the data suggests we only really started to feel the impact of UPFs from 2010 onwards.

It's like filling up a car with poor-quality fuel. You might get down the road a little, but over time, the engine's going to protest and start causing problems.

The biggest issue is this: countries with higher UPF consumption have higher rates of obesity and related diseases than countries where people still eat mostly whole or minimally processed foods.[3]

In the UK, 63% per cent of the population are now overweight or obese. And it's not because we don't exercise enough.[4] This is crazy when you put it into context. Take your ten closest friends. In theory, this means that three of them should be obese, four overweight and three a healthy weight. These are some slap-us-in-the-face and make-us-wake-up numbers.

It is fast becoming clear that it's not just about weight: diets high in UPFs are linked in studies to greater risks of heart disease, type 2 diabetes, certain cancers, depression and more.[5] In the UK, we have some of the leading rates of cancer in the world.

When more than half of everything we eat comes from UPFs, these statistics become very personal. It means your daily packet of crisps and cola isn't just an innocent treat, it's part of a nationwide trend that's literally making us all ill. Something needs to change.

The best place to start is with the weekly food shop. Just watch the items going through at any checkout. Packets of biscuits, flavoured yoghurts, and sliced bread are all the convenient staples of a busy UK life. I used to think that food was just food – if it was sold in supermarkets, it had to be safe, right? Surely the regulators had it covered. How bad could it really be? But the reality is that the biscuits your grandma was buying 50 years ago are not the biscuits you are buying today. We haven't all suddenly become lazy or lacking in willpower, as the media often suggests – the truth is, our food has changed.

Take the ingredients of a biscuit. When it was developed in 1892, the humble digestive was made from the following ingredients and an estimated 16.6% sugar content:

Wheat flour, sugar, malt extract, butter and raising agents.

Today, a Maryland Cookie is 31% sugar (almost double) and has an ingredient list that looks like this:

Wheat flour (wheat flour, calcium carbonate, niacin, iron, thiamin), chocolate chips (25%) (sugar, cocoa mass, vegetable fats (sustainable palm, shea, sal), emulsifiers (soya lecithin, E442, E476), cocoa butter, flavourings), sugar, sustainable palm oil, whey or whey derivatives (milk), partially inverted sugar syrup, raising agents (sodium bicarbonate, ammonium bicarbonate), salt, flavourings.

While it's hard to isolate the exact cause of our poor health outcomes today, it is quite clear that a doubling in sugar content combined with artificial flavourings, emulsifiers and highly processed vegetable fats is a recipe for poor health.

This is a result of commercial decisions made by businesses over decades. If food manufacturers can improve taste, increase shelf life and reduce costs, they are doing their job well commercially speaking. And more often than not, these decisions will be made in a boardroom where health is not a driver.

In fact Big Food has got brilliant at making unhealthy food look healthy. They splash 'high in fibre', 'gluten-free', or 'with vitamins' on the label, while hiding the truth in the ingredients list: ultra-processing, added sugars, and preservatives. Packaging in beautiful shades of green lead us to believe the product is natural and healthy, when it's not. Food manufacturers play into our busy lives, knowing convenience often wins. The sad reality is many of these products are ultra-processed junk, leaving us and our kids hooked on foods that are made with profit in mind.

Is it really food anyway?

Almost all food is processed to some extent because washing, chopping, cooking, and freezing are forms of processing. But processing isn't the villain, it's ULTRA-processing we need to watch out for.

True UPFs are products formulated mostly or entirely from industrial ingredients and additives, with little to no intact whole food remaining. They are edible 'products' that no home cook could ever replicate in their kitchen, because they're made using industrial techniques and contain things you'd never find in a typical pantry.[6]

As one researcher famously put it: 'Most UPF is not food. It's an industrially produced edible substance.'

They are made from cheap ingredients like refined starches, sugars, industrially processed oils, cheap protein powders, and a cocktail of additives like flavour enhancers, colours, sweeteners, emulsifiers, preservatives, thickeners.

Food manufacturers discovered they could make UPFs very cheaply, saving costs because they tend to have an extremely long shelf life. Better still, when you chemically play with food you can tweak the recipe to provide just the perfect amount of sugar, fat and salt, and just the right texture to make them very morish.

A typical UPF ingredient list reads more like a chemistry set than a recipe. Take strawberry yoghurt – a healthy version would contain milk, strawberries, and live cultures. But you can massively extend its shelf life and addictiveness when you remove the fat (so you can give it a healthy label) and add corn starch, carrageenan (a food additive), artificial flavour, and aspartame (a sweetener).

This distinction is important, because it turns out these differences in content and formulation have real consequences for our health.

How UPFs wreck our health

Too many calories:

One of the defining traits of UPFs is that they are engineered to be irresistible. The food industry has perfected recipes that hit our brain chemistry in a certain way, with that perfect combination of salt, sugar, and fat that our brains reward with a surge of pleasure. It's not an accident that you can inhale a whole tube of Pringles or keep refilling your bowl with sugary cereal. These foods are hyper-palatable and often designed to be eaten quickly.

The National Institutes of Health (NIH) in the US demonstrated this dramatically. When people were given ultra-processed meals, they ate on average 500 calories more per day than when they ate unprocessed meals, even though both groups thought they were equally full.[7] In just two weeks, the UPF diet group gained about a kilo of body weight, while the unprocessed group lost weight.

This happens because UPFs tend to be low in fibre and protein, which are macronutrients that fill us up. UPFs also often come in easy-to-munch forms, which means we eat them faster and leave our body's satiety signals lagging behind. They also pack a lot of calories in a small volume – way more than you would find in nature. It's easy to drink 300 calories of orange juice in a minute or two but it's hard to eat 300 calories of oranges in the same time. Ultra-processing essentially strips foods of many natural safeguards against overeating.

Too few nutrients:
People who stock up on UPFs are more likely to be missing out on essential vitamins and minerals along with the lack of protein and fibre. Paradoxically, this can lead to us being overfed calorically yet undernourished biologically.

A study in Australia demonstrated clearly that people who ate UPFs reduced their intake of vitamins A, E, C, B9, B12, zinc, calcium, iron, magnesium, potassium, and phosphorus significantly.[8] That was me: I was rarely hungry, ate full meals, had protein shakes after sport and yet I wasn't getting enough nutrients for my immune system to function properly.

It's all too easy for UPFs to displace more nourishing foods from your life. If a kid is filling up on ultra-processed chicken nuggets for lunch, they're not eating a home-cooked stew that would supply iron and other essential nutrients. Over time, this creates deficiencies – or at least suboptimal health.

Too many additives:

Ultra-processed foods get their taste, texture, and shelf life from a wide range of artificial additives like preservatives, flavourings, artificial sweeteners, emulsifiers, and stabilisers. Regulators generally consider each approved food additive as safe at the levels used. But here's the catch: these approvals are often based on studies that look for acute toxicity or test high doses in isolation, not the cumulative, synergistic effect of eating dozens of different additives, every day, for decades.

No one actually knows what the incremental impact of consuming a bit of sodium nitrite in bacon, some polysorbate-80 in ice cream, a little aspartame in Diet Coke, some artificial red dye in cereal, day in, day out, does to our bodies. But emerging science gives cause for concern.

In a 2015 study, mice that were fed common emusifiers (like carboxymethylcellulose and polysorbate-80) developed chronic inflammation, gained weight, and had altered gut bacteria.[9] While mice aren't humans, the results hint that these additives could be contributing to diseases like inflammatory bowel disease. Other research[10] has linked artificial food dyes to behavioural issues in children, and preservatives like nitrates to promoting cancerous changes (hence the link between processed meat and cancers).[11]

The challenging truth is that the damage from UPFs

often accrues silently over a long period of time. Nobody eats a microwave lasagne and keels over. The health issues linked to UPFs – obesity, diabetes, heart disease, cancer – can typically take 10, 20, 30 years to develop. This slow burn makes it easy for us to ignore the warning signs.

Best to cut back

When a major health problem strikes, it's impossible to say, 'Ah, it was definitely the emulsifiers or the phthalates.' But just because it's hard to prove cause and effect on an individual level, it doesn't mean the cause and effect isn't there – in fact, it's obvious when you look at the macro data on the amount of chronic disease we now have in our society.

This is why I've become passionate about cutting out UPFs in food and other products. By the time the establishment sees unequivocal proof on paper, it might be too late. We've been the guinea pigs in a grand processed-food experiment, and the early results (rising obesity, cancer, heart disease, irritable bowel syndrome etc) are not good. Sure, genetics and lifestyle play a role too, but diet is a common denominator we can control.

Of course, the lines are blurred. Some foods that fall into the UPF category can still contain beneficial nutrients. I know this from my own world – a vitamin tablet is technically ultra-processed, but so long as it contains ONLY vitamins, minerals and natural ingredients, it can still have a positive health outcome, despite the processing.

On the other hand, take a bag of salted crisps. It doesn't classify as a UPF because it only has three ingredients (potatoes, salt and oil), but it's certainly not healthy if you eat a bag every day.

I wrestled with these grey areas for some time, getting frustrated with all the conflicting science and messaging. But I remain true to my beliefs – UPFs are easily identified and, in my experience, best avoided.

After digesting all this information, I believe it is clear: we can't wait for perfect studies or government regulations to do what common sense and our own bodies are already telling us to do – reject ultra-processed foods and other products, as much as we realistically can. This doesn't mean never eat a biscuit or get a takeaway. But it does mean UPFs should no longer be the foundation of our diet; they can be an occasional exception instead.

I encourage you to conduct your own experiment. Don't just take my word – or even the scientists' words – for it – *experience it*. Try cutting out (or cutting down on) ultra-processed foods for a few weeks and see what happens. Notice your energy, your mood, your satiety. You might be surprised at how quickly positive changes come. And remember that while the wheels of science and policy turn slowly, you have agency over your plate in the here and now. The impact of UPFs on blood sugar is especially important, so it's worth diving into this in a bit more detail. Here's the expert view from clinical nutritionist Natalie Burrows.

The lowdown on blood sugar

In recent years, "blood sugar" has moved from medical textbooks into everyday conversation, as growing awareness highlights its role for all of us. Understanding how blood sugars rise and fall throughout the day provides insight into energy fluctuations, concentration, and long-term metabolic health. People are beginning to see that stable blood sugar isn't just a number – it's key for feeling alert, maintaining mood, and supporting overall wellbeing.

Blood sugar, or blood glucose, refers to the amount of glucose circulating in the bloodstream. Glucose is the body's primary energy source, an essential fuel for every cell, and comes mainly from dietary carbohydrates. During digestion, carbohydrates are broken down into simple sugars, including glucose, which then enter the bloodstream. The body regulates this process carefully through hormones, chiefly insulin, which enables cells to absorb glucose for energy use or storage.

Yet the importance of blood sugar goes far beyond providing energy. The brain alone consumes about 60% of the body's glucose supply in fasted, resting states, highlighting how crucial it is for clear thinking, mood, and daily functioning. While both very high (hyperglycaemia) and very low (hypoglycaemia) blood sugar can be harmful, it is the chronic elevation of blood sugar that drives many of today's major health challenges.

At the heart of this lies insulin resistance, a state where the body's cells no longer respond effectively to insulin's signal to allow glucose in, leaving it to accumulate in the blood. This is a key step on the path towards type 2 diabetes and other metabolic disorders – a health concern projected to rise by 25% by

2030 and by more than 50% by 2045, affecting hundreds of millions worldwide and profoundly impacting quality of life.

A key factor under the spotlight for the steep rise in metabolic issues is our modern food environment. Studies have shown that high ultra-processed food (UPF) intake is associated with increased risk of chronic health conditions. UPFs now make up more than half of the calories consumed in many Western diets. These foods are designed for taste and convenience but are often stripped of adequate fibre, while remaining high in refined starches, added sugars, and unhealthy fats. They are highly palatable foods and therefore easier to over-consume.

The solution is not to fear carbohydrates or strive for rigid control, but to make conscious swaps. Wholefood sources of carbohydrates, such as vegetables, beans, legumes, fruit, and minimally processed darker wholegrains, provide fibre, vitamins, minerals, and phytonutrients that support balanced blood sugar responses and benefit overall health. Balanced meals that combine protein, healthy fats, and fibre-rich carbo-hydrates help avoid sharp blood sugar highs and the potential lows that follow, keeping energy and concentration steady.

Although blood sugar may seem like a minor detail in the broader picture of health, it underpins much of how we feel and function daily. In today's world of convenience-driven eating, understanding it can be one of the most powerful steps we can take toward achieving lasting energy, improved cognition, and good metabolic health.

Natalie Louise Burrows
Registered clinical nutritionist and clinic director of Integral Wellness, a cardiometabolic health and nutrition clinic

Ultra-processed ON your body too

There's plenty of science to support my fears about putting too many chemicals into our bodies, but in the quest for optimal health I believe it's important to have a big, long think about the chemical load you add to that through personal care and cleaning products, and to have that in mind when you're putting those extra items in your shopping trolley.

When there are chemical nasties in toothpaste, deodorants, shampoos, sunscreens and household cleaners it makes sense to steer clear of some of them if you can.

Take a glance at the back of a bottle of shampoo or kitchen cleaner today and you'll find the ingredients read more like a laboratory list than something you'd find in your cupboards at home. But it wasn't always this way. In the 1960s, most household and personal care products contained just a handful of simple ingredients. Shampoo might have been little more than soap flakes and herbal extracts; cleaning sprays often relied on vinegar, lemon juice and bicarbonate of soda.

Fast forward 60 years and those same products have become ever more complex, packed with surfactants, foaming agents, stabilisers, preservatives, synthetic fragrances, and colourants. The results are undeniably effective, delivering spotless bathrooms, glossy hair, and fresh smells on demand.

Just as with food, the question isn't whether these products work, it's what the long-term accumulation of all those additives might be doing to us.

Let's take soap as an example:

1960s soap ingredients:
Tallow (animal fat) or vegetable oils (e.g. olive oil, coconut oil), lye (sodium hydroxide), water, natural essential oil for fragrance.

Today's shower gel ingredients:
Water, sodium laureth sulfate (synthetic foaming agent), cocamidopropyl betaine (secondary surfactant), glycerin (humectant), PEG-7 glyceryl cocoate (emulsifier), sodium chloride (thickener), phenoxyethanol, methylparaben, propylparaben (preservatives), parfum (synthetic fragrance, often a blend of dozens of chemicals), CI 42090 / CI 14720 (artificial colours), citric acid (pH adjuster), disodium EDTA (stabiliser, prevents soap scum in hard water).

That's 10+ ingredients – many synthetic, designed for foaming, fragrance, stability, and shelf life. The end product might look and smell appealing, but it's a far cry from the humble soap bars of the past.

As with UPFs, official regulators deem each ingredient safe at the levels used, but what no one really knows is the effect that absorbing dozens of these compounds over many years could be having.

We know we can absorb chemicals through our skin (otherwise hormone replacement therapy and nicotine patches wouldn't work), so how many of these chemicals end up in our bodies? Inevitably, some people will be more sensitive than others. People who suffer from eczema or allergies, for example, often notice the effects first.

I'm not suggesting a dramatic return to the Dark Ages, but it is worth remembering that aluminium-free deodorants, natural shampoos, and vinegar-based cleaners often work just as well – and in many cases cost no more than – their ultra-processed equivalents.

Ultra-processed environment

It isn't just our health at stake; ultra-processed cleaning and personal care products also take a heavy toll on the environment. Did you know that in 1974 the world produced just 2 million tonnes of plastic packaging a year? Today that figure is closer to 140 million tonnes, with less than 10% ever being recycled. Most of it ends up in landfills or oceans, where it slowly breaks down into microplastics. And plastics aren't neutral: the very additives that make them flexible, colourful, or durable leach into soil and water as they degrade.

Synthetic fragrances and surfactants have been detected in rivers and lakes around the world, altering the behaviour and reproduction of wildlife. Much like UPFs, these products have been engineered for convenience and profit, but the hidden costs of pollution, chemical accumulation and ecosystem disruption are quietly mounting in the background.

The good news is that swapping out plastic-heavy liquid shampoos for solid shampoo bars, choosing biodegradable cleaning sprays, or buying refillable bottles instead of single-use plastics are all simple changes that are all readily available in your local supermarket.

Finding 'healthy' between the 'good' and the 'bad'

In a world saturated with one-size-fits-all health advice, there's a quiet but powerful truth that often gets overlooked: your health journey is yours alone. It doesn't start with a perfect diet plan, a punishing workout routine, or the latest trend in wellness. It starts with one simple, intentional step… one that reflects who you are, where you're starting from, and what matters most to you.

How are you feeling about your health today?

Where are you in your life right now, where do you want to be and how much time and energy do you have to commit to a healthier you?

The answers to these questions will tell you exactly how far and how fast you need to go. I appreciate everyone has their own unique set of pressures and priorities. This book is about giving you the tools to make positive changes to your health, as small or as large as they need to be.

Whether you're a complete beginner trying to get moving again, someone managing a chronic condition, a parent juggling multiple priorities, or an athlete looking to fine-tune your performance, your needs are unique, and your next step will be within this book.

There's a common misconception that getting healthy requires a dramatic overhaul. But the truth is, sustainable health is built through small, consistent actions that add up over time. Whether it's choosing water over juice, walking instead of taking the lift, or getting an extra hour of sleep, these little decisions are all that matter. The best health journeys are built on realistic, compassionate advice that honours your life context.

This is the fundamental message behind the concept of *The Good, the Bad, and the Healthy*. You don't have to strive to be good and worry about falling short. It is enough to know where 'good' is, and what's 'bad' (this might sometimes surprise you!); my quest in this book is to show you the many ways to be a little more 'healthy' with the options which sit between those two extremes.

We all live busy lives, we all have budgetary constraints, and doing our best is more than enough.

Small changes, big impact

Change is hard. We've all had that burst of motivation to overhaul our diet on Monday, only to find that, by Friday, the kale has wilted and we've given into our guilty pleasure again.

One reason small swaps work is that they slip under the radar of our internal resistance. Trading your white bread for brown or swapping to a healthier yoghurt shouldn't feel like a massive sacrifice – but you'll be getting a burst of extra nutrients and balancing your blood sugar levels. Switching chemical deodorant for a natural stick deodorant might mean you notice your armpits smell different, but your body will register the drop in compounds being absorbed through your skin and adapt.

Rather than going all 'healthy' and cutting out your favourite foods and personal care items, it's easy to just make a few mini switches that are easy to stick to and don't leave you feeling deprived or punished.

There's robust science to support the benefit of making small changes. It's all about 'compound growth', which is a principle well-known in the finance world and equally powerful when applied to our daily habits.

Striving to improve your health and habits by just 1% each day may seem insignificant – in fact, you might barely register the change. For instance, take the 'five-a-day' vegetable target. One portion is about 80g, so five portions means about 400g of vegetables a day. Increasing that by 1% just means adding an extra 4g – which is 15 extra peas or sweetcorn kernels, or a thin slice of apple. It's nothing!

But if you accumulate enough 'one percents' in the things you buy – just one or two from different aisles of the supermarket as you do your shopping – the gains will start to mount. Stick with these swaps for a year, and those tiny gains will add up to something astonishing, with health benefits layering on top of health benefits and multiplying as they accumulate.

The maths on this is mind-blowing. If you aim to make a 1%-sized change every day for a year, you won't be 365% healthier 12 months later, you'll be 3,678% heathier. This is because each day's improvement builds on top of all the previous improvements and compounds.

As author James Clear puts it, "making a choice that is 1% better or 1% worse seems insignificant in the moment, but over the span of moments that make up a lifetime, these choices determine the difference between who you are and who you could be."[12]

The grand overhaul that only lasts a week can't compete with small improvements sustained over many months.

A key element of the 1%-better approach is focusing on progress, not perfection. Nobody lives the perfect life 365 days of the year. Progress doesn't get upset if you have a cheat meal, it doesn't tut-tut at the beer you drank last night. Progress simply says, 'In what ways can you be 1% healthier than you currently are?'

Giving yourself permission to not be perfect and to improve in micro-steps is fundamental to shifting your health sustainably in the long-term. If yesterday you had a bag of crisps with lunch, pick a healthier bag of crisps today – one that's baked not fried. Easy. Then, as you get comfortable with that, why not try swapping the baked crisps for salted nuts? These have more good fats and protein than your typical bag of crisps, and will fill you up for longer. Once you've nailed that, maybe you can swap from the fried salted nuts to raw nuts that aren't fried?

The idea is to upgrade your choices in a way that feels easy and satisfying, and to maintain the spirit of what you enjoy but upgrade the quality.

Love a fry-up breakfast? Keep the eggs and mushrooms but consider swapping the white toast for sourdough and the fried hash browns for a slice of avocado. Enjoy pasta for dinner? Have your spaghetti but swap half the pasta for extra courgettes in the sauce and you'll painlessly eat more veg and slightly less refined starch.

Over weeks and months, these small improvements lead to an eating pattern that is much higher in nutrients, fibre, and wholefoods, and lower in added sugar and unhealthy ultra-processed ingredients.

And the best part of it all is: by approaching it gradually, your taste buds and cravings adjust along the way. Taste bud cells regenerate approximately every 10 to 14 days, so you might be surprised that after a while you will actually prefer the sourdough bread or find the Greek yoghurt with real strawberries more satisfying than the flavoured kind. That's when you know these swaps have become a true habit that you will stick to for the rest of your life.

The same principle applies to non-food purchases too. That new natural toothpaste may have a weird taste at first, but within a couple of weeks, it'll be the only thing your taste buds know.

Rely on habits, not willpower

Why do these tiny swaps work when grand resolutions so often fail? The magic lies in how our brains form habits and make decisions. Turning small swaps into long-term habits is something psychologists call "habit stacking". This technique involves linking a new desired behaviour onto an existing habit or cue, so the two become connected in your daily routine.

Stanford behavioural scientist BJ Fogg, known for his work on tiny habits, suggests that the key to making a habit stick is to make it easy and tie it to a trigger that's already stable in your life.[13] In practice, this could look like: "After I make my morning coffee, I'll eat a piece of fruit", or, "When I sit down for my usual evening TV show, I'll grab a bowl of nuts so I fill up and don't want to snack on something else."

The existing habit (making coffee or watching TV) acts as the anchor. It's something you reliably do every day and, by intentionally following it with the new small swap, you take advantage of the momentum of the old routine. Over time, the new behaviour latches on and becomes an automatic part of that old routine. Habit stacking works especially well for food swaps because eating tends to have built-in routines (like mealtimes or snack times) that you can piggyback on.

Research on habit formation has shown that repetition in a consistent context is key. On average, it takes about 66 days for a new habit to become automatic, though this can vary from person to person, and a recent 2025 study found that it can take up to a year to really establish and embed one into your life.[14,15] Researchers found that success can be influenced by how frequently you undertake the new activity (e.g. it's better to make the change every day rather than just two days a week), and the timing of the practice (e.g. making it part of something you already do every day like brushing your teeth). And, of course, the particularly important bit is to make the habit something you enjoy, which can feed into your swaps – they don't have to be joyless!

The 1%-better philosophy can transform other areas of your life too. Often, success in one domain spills over into others. When you see how effective small changes in your food can be, you might feel inspired to apply the same approach elsewhere. For example, you could start taking the stairs instead of the lift at work (a small activity swap that boosts fitness) or commit to powering down screens one hour earlier at night (a tiny change for better sleep).

If 10k steps a day seems an insurmountable hurdle, is it easier to think that 1% is just 100 steps? And if you really can't get your head around going to bed an hour earlier, know that 1% of an hour is just 36 seconds. You'll be doubling your 1% target if you set a new bedtime just one minute earlier each night!

The beauty is that it's all interconnected: eating a bit healthier gives you more energy, which might make you more inclined to take that short evening walk; sleeping better improves your willpower the next day, which might make sticking to your food swaps easier, and so on. Each positive habit makes the next one a tad easier, creating an upward spiral of wellness.

Just as the old saying goes, look after the pennies and the pounds will take care of themselves. Calories saved or nutrients added gradually can transform your health profile. You might not see changes tomorrow or next week, but give it a few months and your jeans will fit a bit looser, and your energy levels will climb. The best part is, you're not on a "diet" rollercoaster; you're simply living a healthier life.

So go ahead and celebrate the small wins. Cook one more homemade dinner this week than you did last week and acknowledge the progress. Or cook one element of the meal from scratch. Every little counts.

Your journey is not linear

Progress is rarely a straight line. Some days you'll feel strong and motivated; others, tired or discouraged. Life brings interruptions, challenges, and curveballs. But the important thing is to stay engaged with your journey, even – and most importantly – when it feels messy or imperfect. Only then can you learn to listen to your body and trust yourself more each day.

Too often, health is reduced to numbers: weight, body mass index, calories, steps. But true health encompasses much more. It's not just how your body looks, but how it functions. It's not just the absence of illness, but the presence of joy and purpose. Success, then, is not about reaching some arbitrary ideal. It's about becoming the healthiest, most fulfilled version of you. And only you can define what that looks like.

Go at your own pace, one step at a time. Try one of my healthy swaps, then add more when you're ready, and keep stacking them up.

No matter where you're starting from, whether you feel like you're thriving, surviving, or somewhere in between, your health journey starts now. Not tomorrow. Not when everything is perfect. *Now.*

So ask yourself: what's one small thing I can do today that moves me toward better health? Pick a page – and start from there.

From my health journey to yours, I hope this helps.

SUPERMARKET SWAPS

FRUIT AND VEGETABLES

When you walk into any large supermarket, the first area you have to navigate is usually the fruit and veg section. If you're tired, distracted, stressed and feeling the financial pinch, this can be a minefield. So many colours, varieties, packages and not a scooby what you're going to be cooking this week. It's no wonder you have no idea where to start.

This is often the hardest part of the weekly shop. In those first stressful minutes, you've got to try to figure out what vegetable you need to make that meal on Thursday night; how many will you need? Will they last until the weekend without going mushy?

Vegetables and fruit are probably the single most important items in your shopping trolley, yet only 33% of us actually manage to hit the five portions a day recommended by the UK health authorities.[16] It's just too easy to think of fruits and veg as time-consuming to prepare, expensive, unpopular with the kids, and far too likely to end up rotting at the back of the fridge.

These are the barriers we need to overcome to make sure we eat more. I don't need to tell you what the science says about how healthy they are. It doesn't matter what you pick up in these aisles, you'll be getting important vitamins, polyphenols (anti-inflammatory plant compounds) and fibre.

My job is to make it easier for you to consume more

of them. And if you are ready to eat more, let's get stuck into the detail about how you optimise the habit for your health.

Let's make it simple:

THE GOOD
Seasonal, UK-grown, maybe organic

THE BAD
Out-of-season produce, shipped from far-flung locations

THE HEALTHY
Everything fruit and veg is healthy.
Fill your trolley!

Here's how to nudge the healthy upwards when you shop for fruit and vegetables

1. Think seasonal

The first easy win is to aim for seasonal produce. This means choosing strawberries in June, July and August, runner beans in September, and root veg like parsnips in the winter months. Seasonal fruits and veg tend to be cheaper when they are in season as they are readily available and there is a surplus in the market. We've got used to picking up our favourites all year round, but start checking the packs – has that asparagus been shipped from Kenya, or those beans from Peru?

The logistics and costs of importing fruit and veg from the other side of the world drive up the price. If you're flying cherry tomatoes in from Morocco in the middle of January, there are environmental costs to consider too.

Buying UK produce at roughly the time of year that it is naturally grown and harvested will not only save money and reduce your carbon footprint, but also boost your health.

Why would a strawberry grown locally be healthier? Simple. Age. The fresher the fruit the more nutrients it packs. A strawberry grown in Kent could reach the supermarket in 1-2 days from picking. In the winter, on a lorry from Spain, it may take 5-7 days for that strawberry to reach your shelf. And while they do *look* fresh on the shelf, vitamins like C and B, and other antioxidants, start to degrade the moment they are picked.

Fresh fruits and vegetables are also usually picked before peak ripeness to allow them to ripen during the long journey to reach your local supermarket. This gives them less time to develop the full range of vitamins, minerals and natural antioxidants they'd get if they were left longer to ripen in the field.

2. Add variety

The vast populations of microbes that live in our gut thrive on variety, and if we feed them a wide range of different types of fruit and vegetables, they reward us by pumping out chemicals that improve our mood, our immunity and so many other beneficial aspects of our health. So don't get stuck in a fruit and vegetable rut, reaching for the same selection every single time you go shopping. Aim to pick up something unfamiliar and new each time you're at the supermarket.

3. *Get a nutrient boost*

If you are looking to optimise your nutrient and polyphenol content, here are some healthier swaps to get you started:

SWAPS

White onion → Red onion
For higher polyphenols and quercetin.

Iceberg lettuce → Romaine
For higher vitamin K, folate and antioxidants.

White mushrooms → Chestnut mushrooms
For higher antioxidants.

Banana → Kiwi
For more vitamin C, vitamin K and fibre.

As a rule of thumb, the darker the fruit or veg, the higher the polyphenol count. Even within apple varieties, a dark red Royal Gala apple will have more nutrients per gram than a Golden Delicious.

4. *When to choose organic*

Does organic matter? Does it make fruits or vegetables healthier? The short answer is yes AND no. No one wants to get a mouthful of pesticides when they're chewing on a pear, but an organic label doesn't technically make the fruit healthier from a nutritional standpoint.

Personally, I try to pick out the organic options whenever I can. But I appreciate it is more expensive and, for some, that makes it out of reach. So, the simple trick is to follow the 'Clean Fifteen' and 'Dirty Dozen' list. These are official lists, which rank the 15 types of fruit and vegetable crops most likely to be free from pesticides and the 12 most likely to have pesticide residue left on them when you bring them home. The 'dirty' ones are usually those that are more heavily sprayed and treated with pesticides as they grow.

In the simplest terms, if non-organic is kind of 'bad' and organic is 'good' (in an ideal world), then at least you know you'll be 'healthy' by choosing ordinary non-organic if you're buying from the Clean Fifteen list and you can decide whether you want to pay extra for organic when you're picking up something from the Dirty Dozen.

Clean: Avocados, sweetcorn, pineapples, cabbages, peas, onions, asparagus, mangoes, papayas, kiwis, aubergines, grapefruits, melons, cauliflowers, sweet potatoes

Dirty: Strawberries, spinach, kale and spring greens, grapes, peaches, pears, nectarines, apples, peppers, cherries, blueberries, green beans.[17]

Another way to simply avoid the pesticides that we know aren't great for our health is to properly wash your fruit and veg. A rinse under the tap might not be enough — try filling a bowl of water, adding a teaspoon of bicarbonate of soda and giving them a dunk, then rinse.

5. Just eat more

It's up to you how far you go with this and how much you choose to invest in your health, but the simple takeaway is to create ways in your daily life to eat more fruit and vegetables. Your body will thank you. Alongside all the vitamins, minerals, polyphenols and antioxidants you are getting from your increase in consumption, you will also be benefitting from the extra fibre, which will support your gut health too. You may think this isn't you – but 9 in 10 people in the UK do not consume enough fibre daily – so we are all in this together.[18]

How to eat more fruit and veg

- **Add fruit and veg to EVERYTHING!** Throw two kinds of fruit on your yoghurt in the morning. Add an avocado and tomatoes to your lunch, or try to add at least three veg to any dinner-time meal. You'll be on seven-a-day before even thinking about an apple for a snack.

- **Put them where you least expect it.** Did you know you can make pasta with courgettes, cake with carrots, and even pancakes with banana? Fruit and veg can be the insanely versatile base for any dish. Stop thinking traditionally and start being creative.

- **Bring back the classic meat and two veg**. This was how everyone cooked in England in the 1950s and it's a tradition we've lost a little since our recipes have become more international, but it really is a fundamental way to think about the make-up of your plate.

These are just three tools I use to incorporate more fruit and veg in my life. You'll find more inspiration in my chapters on the freezer section and tinned food too.

It's not always easy and it's not always achievable, but don't worry about that. We can't be perfect all the time. What matters is eating a bit more fruit and veg than you do right now. Some days will be easier than others.

BREAD

Ahhh, the sweet smell of freshly baked bread in the bakery aisle – something that evokes childhood memories for me of camping trips in France and venturing out early every morning to pick up a fresh baguette from the local bakery.

Bread is something we all know and love, and the supermarket bakery aisle is bursting with choices, usually presented as a wall of plastic-wrapped squishiness: white, brioche, wholemeal, seeded, high in fibre, sliced, pittas, wraps, rolls and bagels. It can be quite overwhelming.

Here's the lowdown:

THE GOOD
Proper sourdough with 4-5 ingredients.

THE BAD
Ultra-processed white bread, rolls and wraps with long lists of ingredients and an impossibly long shelf life.

THE HEALTHY
Wholegrain unprocessed bread products with a short list of ingredients.

The worry is that cheap sliced bread, and all those other plastic-wrapped bread products, are packed with chemical additives and preservatives. Did you know that the way bread is made can completely change how your body digests it? The production process can even make certain nutrients more bioavailable, yet typical ultra-processed bread contains few of these goodies and instead has upwards of 20 ingredients plus added sugar. Even your supposedly healthy wholemeal seeded sliced loaf is packed with preservatives and emulsifiers. Added seeds bring nutrients and fibre, but it is unfortunate that the corporate machine has adulterated the recipe for palatability and shelf life.

So, what do we do? Where do we start? There are levels to the bread game. First off, let's settle the white vs brown debate. Essentially, white flour is stripped of the bran and germ of the wheat to give it its milky-white appearance, which is purely cosmetic. The problem is, the bits that are removed contain most of the fibre, vitamins and minerals. So as a first step in the healthy direction, wholemeal is always higher in fibre and better for your health.

A great way to avoid UPFs in the bread aisle is to always look for the traditional classic breads that haven't been messed with. Think pittas, bake-at-home baguettes and ciabattas, which stick to their authentic recipes and have far fewer additives (you can do a quick check of the ingredients to confirm this). That way you can cut the junk but still enjoy the aisle with freedom.

The beauty of bread is its versatility. It comes in different shapes, sizes and styles for any occasion and there are plenty of better choices on offer than the typical UPF white sliced. Dark rye bread is a great example of a healthy bread that hasn't been modified. Sure, it's a bit of an acquired taste, but it is usually available everywhere and it toasts really well.

Try these swaps:

SWAPS

Bagels → Pittas
For an affordable daily staple that isn't UPF.

Wraps/tortillas → Italian wraps
Made with olive oil and fewer additives.

White baguettes → Ciabattas
For added olive oil and fewer ingredients.

Many people reach for a bagel as a lunch staple. Unfortunately, I'm yet to find a clean-label bagel in the supermarkets, which is why I suggest the swap to pittas. But I'm sure if you head online or to your local bakery there are some "better-for-you" bagels out there if you just can't give them up.

All hail sourdough

Sourdough stands out because, when made properly, it contains no additives, preservatives or seed oils. Unlike factory breads, which are loaded with processing agents, sourdough's simpler method keeps it closer to wholefood status.

Sourdough is one of the oldest breads in the world, dating back over 5,000 years to ancient Egypt, when bakers relied on naturally occurring wild yeasts and bacteria to ferment their dough long before commercial yeast was invented.

Sourdough's slow fermentation process enhances its digestibility, as the fermentation helps produce prebiotics, which feed the beneficial bacteria in your gut, supporting long-term digestive and immune health. Some people with mild gluten sensitivities (though not full coeliac disease) also find sourdough easier to digest, because fermentation partially breaks down those gluten molecules.

The fermentation process that makes sourdough creates a complexity in the bread that helps lower its glycaemic index (54 compared to a conventional loaf at 71), helping to slow blood sugar release.

Another often overlooked benefit is that sourdough bread contains about 40% less sugar per 100 grams than most breads. This reduction in sugar may not seem much – as there is only typically 3.5g per two slices of regular shop bread – but savings can soon add up. Assuming you have two slices of toast for breakfast and lunch, you would be cutting 2.8g of sugar a day. Over a year that's a whole kilo of sugar slashed from your diet. The cut in sugar is not just good news for our waistlines but also for our overall health, contributing to a balanced diet without the same spikes in blood sugar levels.

Whilst most of us tend to think of sourdough as a weekend brunch treat, perhaps with eggs and avocado, it's become a surprisingly affordable staple in most major supermarkets now. Bread is something most people consume every single day and changing to sourdough can have a huge and exponential health benefit over the years.

You can now find real sourdough in most of the major supermarkets. To spot authentic sourdough, check the ingredients list. It should only include flour, water, salt, and a starter. Avoid loaves with added yeast, sugar, or vinegar as they are not likely to be fermented authentically.

My recommendations are:

- Tesco Brown Sourdough
- ASDA Extra Special White Sourdough (although this has added rapeseed oil – more on this later)
- Sainsbury's Sourdough Pave, Taste the Difference
- Waitrose No.1 White Sourdough Bread
- Morrisons – currently doesn't have an own-label loaf, but they do stock Jason's The Great White Straight Up Sourdough

Yes, sourdough is more expensive, but you are only likely to be spending around 20-30% more per loaf, which over the course of a year (assuming a loaf a week) is a small extra outlay for a stronger gut microbiome, more nutrients and less sugar. Something I think is well worth the investment.

Gluten-free

It's worth adding a note on the gluten-free options that have exploded into the supermarket over the last decade. These might be great if you're coeliac because your options are so limited, but not to be recommended if you can tolerate some gluten.

The problem is, it is hard to make bread products with gluten-free flour, so numerous artificial additives have to be thrown in to improve the taste and mouth feel. That means GF loaves and wraps are extremely ultra-processed, with long lists of ingredients including starches, gums, and added sugar. They're often lower in fibre and nutrients than standard bread too.

A better option for many people who are sensitive to gluten – if you're not coeliac – is authentic sourdough, which can be easier to digest thanks to the long fermentation process which helps to break down the gluten without getting rid of it completely. Anyone with any kind of serious gluten sensitivity should avoid it and it most definitely is not safe for those with coeliac disease. If you do need to eat a gluten-free diet, seek out brands with shorter, simpler ingredients lists. Some of the best gluten-free options are often foods that wouldn't contain any gluten anyway!

SWAPS

GF wraps → Corn tortillas
Naturally gluten-free, simpler recipe.

GF crackers → Oat cakes
Fewer additives.

GF Pasta → Lentil pasta
Higher in protein and fibre than typical GF options.

MILK

We all have milk in the fridge, but there's long been debate about the healthiest kind of milk to put in your cup of tea or coffee. On average, Brits drink over 62 litres per year, so it's worth getting this choice right.[19] In recent years, oat milk has soared up the popularity charts, thanks to its plant-based, environmentally friendly health halo.

But it might surprise you that, despite all the flack about dietary fat, cow's milk is probably one of the greatest sources of nutrition in the British diet. It's the density of essential nutrients per calorie and our high consumption rate that make milk such a core part of our nutrition.

The fascinating truth is that not all milk is created equal. While most of us run through the supermarket grabbing a carton of semi-skimmed as we fly past the chiller aisle, a closer look at how milk is produced reveals some important differences that are worth considering when you're thinking about making your daily swaps.

In a nutshell:

THE GOOD
Full-fat cow's milk delivers calcium, protein, and essential vitamins (ideally organic).

THE BAD
Sweetened plant milks come with a long list of ingredients often including added sugars, oils, and thickeners.

> **THE HEALTHY**
> If you can tolerate dairy products, go for full-fat dairy (organic if you can afford it), and unhomogenised if you can find it. If you're plant-based or lactose-intolerant, go for unsweetened, unprocessed almond or coconut milk.

Whole vs low fat

For years, we were told to choose skimmed or semi-skimmed milk to cut down on the fat in our diets. But the science now tells a different story – whole milk is the most complete and nutritious choice. It contains around 3.6% fat, which makes it more satiating and, importantly, the fat is what stores a lot of the nutrition in milk such as the vitamins A, D, E and K. These nutrients are crucial for immune function, bone health and even hormone balance.

Nutrient	Role	Found in full-fat?	Found in skimmed?
Vitamin A	Vision, immunity, skin health	✔ High	✘ Almost none
Vitamin D	Bone health, immunity	✔ Present	✘ Usually removed unless added back in
Vitamin E	Antioxidant	✔ Yes	✘ Negligible
Vitamin K2	Heart & bone health	✔ Trace amounts	✘ Very low

Homogenised vs unhomogenised

Remember that creamy few inches you'd get at the top of a milk bottle back in the day? Where did it go? Sadly, we lost it due to a process called homogenisation. Almost all milk you find on the supermarket shelves is now homogenised, which means it is processed so that the fat molecules stay evenly mixed throughout, giving it a consistent texture, as apparently that's what we prefer. But studies[20] show how this process may also alter how fat is absorbed within the body. Normally, milk fat exists as large globules surrounded by a natural membrane. When milk is homogenised, these globules are broken down into very tiny particles, which increases their surface area. Some researchers believe this could alter the way fats interact with the gut and bloodstream, potentially leading to faster absorption and a different metabolic response compared to unhomogenised milk. That's why I tend to lean towards old-fashioned unhomogenised milk if I can. While more traditional and slightly harder to find, it's the more wholefood version of milk and is closer to what our grandparents drank. It's not a deal breaker, but it's something I always look out for in the supermarket.

A2 milk (Jersey/Guernsey) vs normal milk

Most supermarket milk comes from Holstein cows and contains a type of protein called A1 beta-casein, which some people find hard to digest. By contrast, Jersey and Guernsey cows produce milk with more of a different type of protein called A2 beta-casein, which is gentler on the digestive system and less likely to cause bloating. So, if you find yourself feeling a bit bloated after drinking milk, it's worth trying Jersey milk as an alternative.

Organic vs non-organic

Is organic worth the extra money? This is a question I get asked all the time. The answer is: it depends on the product. In the case of organic milk, studies have shown that it often contains higher levels of omega-3 fats and slightly more antioxidants, due to the fact that cows reared organically tend to spend more of their life eating grass and less time indoors eating grain.[21] Yes, organic milk costs a bit more – roughly 35% – but for a product most people consume daily, I think it's a relatively small health investment for great nutritional gains.

Pasteurisation: the safety step

Pasteurisation is a separate heat step that knocks out harmful bugs and makes milk safe to drink – pretty much all shop-bought milk is pasteurised. Raw (unpasteurised) milk can carry pathogens like E. coli, Salmonella and Listeria, so public health advice is to stick with pasteurised milk, especially for children, pregnant women, older adults and anyone with a weakened immune system. In the UK, raw milk must carry a safety warning and isn't recommended for vulnerable groups.

SWAPS

Semi-skimmed → Full-fat
For more nutrition and less processing.

> **Homogenised → Unhomogenised milk**
> To make your milk easier to digest and less processed.
>
> **Standard cow's milk → A2 Jersey/Guernsey milk**
> Easier on digestion thanks to A2 protein.

Plant-based milk

When you put a carton of plant-based milk in your shopping trolley you probably have health and sustainability in mind. But the assumption that just because a product comes from plants it must be healthy is an over-simplified one. I had my time with plant-based milks as it was all the rage, and we all leant into the idea of saving the planet by cutting back on dairy consumption, but as I've dug deeper into the research, my views have changed.

Let's break down the nuances of plant-based milks to help you make the healthiest choice:

The Classic – soy milk: The veteran in the plant milk space, soy milk stands tall with its high protein content at 3.4g per 100ml and low sugars (only 0.5g per 100ml). But soy milk does contain isoflavones, which are natural compounds that can weakly mimic oestrogen in the body. While this has sparked concerns about hormonal effects, especially in men, the science is clear: moderate soy consumption doesn't lower testosterone or harm fertility. The rare negative effects you might read about? They usually come from people drinking *litres* of soy milk every day. You're unlikely to see any impact if you're just splashing it in your morning coffee. Find a brand with a short ingredients list (soya beans and water) to avoid unnecessary chemical additives.

The Verdict: Enjoy occasionally, but not in everything.

The Sustainability Champion – oat milk: Oat milk has seduced us all with its creamy texture and eco-friendly footprint. However, it's hiding a sugary secret: the starchy nature of this delicious liquid means it packs 3.4g of sugar per 100ml. Put that in your daily latte and you'll be drinking over 10g of sugar you didn't know you were having per day – that's well over 3kg of extra sugar a year. I know it tastes good, but that's a lot of sugar worth avoiding.

The Verdict: Time to find a new alternative.

The Nutty One – almond milk: Light and with a delicate nutty flavour, almond milk is a low-sugar charmer perfect for the calorie-conscious because it contains only 15kcal and 0g of sugar per 100ml. That's 4x lower in calories than oat milk and 10g less sugar per latte. A small swap with a huge impact.

The Verdict: Your new BFF for health.

The Exotic One – coconut milk: With its tropical taste and light consistency, coconut milk is a favourite in cooking and baking. It is rich in medium-chain triglycerides (MCTs), which is a healthy fat that can support metabolism. And it is a lower-sugar alternative too. This is a great option but watch out for additives like thickeners and gums.

The Verdict: Good to go without the additives, so read the label.

When you are navigating the sea of options in this sector, the big thing to remember is to keep an eye on the ingredients list, as many plant milks are packed with hidden additives. Find the shortest ingredients list you can. You'd think coconut milk would be made from coconut flesh and water, but take a look at the label on the back of one leading brands:

Water, coconut milk [5.7%] [coconut cream [2.6%]], water, hulled soya beans [2.9%], sugar, fructose, acidity regulators [potassium phosphates], calcium [calcium carbonate], sea salt, flavouring, stabiliser [gellan gum].[22]

It's the same for other plant milks too. The best plant-based milk looks like this:

Spring water, organic almonds 5%, Sea Salt.[23]

SWAPS

Processed plant milks → Non-UPF plant milks
For fewer additives, oils and sugars.

Oat lattes → Almond lattes
To cut 9-10 grams of hidden sugar per cup
(over 3kg a year).

Flavoured plant milks → Plain unsweetened versions
Skip the vanilla, chocolate, and barista blends, which are often loaded with extras you don't want.

The good news is there is little variance in price, so you can choose a milk to suit your health and taste preferences best. My recommendation is to invest in a premium brand like Plenish. Its almond milk is typically only around 10–20% more than branded oat drinks – a small uplift for a cleaner, minimally processed recipe with no added gums or oils and a higher nut content.

YOGHURT

Stop by the yoghurt aisle and you'll be bombarded with choices. Such variety and versatility – this sea of pots, cartons and snack tubes ensures that there is something for everyone. But don't be fooled – they are not all as healthy as they seem.

Back in the 1990s, Big Food played a dirty health trick on us all with the invention of zero-fat yoghurt, created to meet demand during the low-fat food craze. Yoghurts were cleverly reformulated to strip out the fat so you could tuck into a low-calorie fat-free chilled dessert without feeling guilty or putting on weight – in theory. The problem? Without fat, yoghurt tastes bland and thin. So manufacturers found a solution by adding loads of sugar, starches, stabilisers, artificial sweeteners, and flavourings to make their chemically enhanced dairy product palatable.

The irony is that in chasing 'healthier' low-fat options, they ended up with a distinctly unhealthy ultra-processed product, which makes a mockery of the health halo that hovers over the dairy aisle.

Thankfully, the science of nutrition today has moved on and dairy fats are NOT to be feared anymore. For decades, dietary fat was pulled out as the primary cause of heart disease, but we now know that sugar is a far bigger culprit. Not all fats are equal, and dairy fat doesn't behave the way we were led to believe. Zero-fat is certainly not the best option. Studies now show that full-fat dairy products are not linked to higher heart disease risk, and in some cases may even be protective.

> **THE GOOD**
> Authentic strained natural Greek yoghurt, which is a great source of protein and provides probiotics for gut health, and calcium for strong bones.
>
> **THE BAD**
> Zero-fat flavoured yoghurts with a long list of chemical ingredients.
>
> **THE HEALTHY**
> Plain full-fat yoghurt, or pots with real fruit pieces and a handful of ingredients.

What's so good about Greek?

Greek yoghurt is thicker and creamier than other varieties because it is made by fermenting yoghurt in tanks and then straining out the liquid during the final steps. The process results in a product with a higher protein content and less sugar.

Greek yoghurt has been eaten for over 2,000 years, with roots in ancient Greece, where it was prized for its rich texture and nourishing qualities. It is still a staple all over the country, including in places like Ikaria, one of the world's 'Blue Zones' where record numbers of people live into their 90s and beyond.

But here's the truth – not all Greek yoghurt is created in the traditional way; you have to watch out for Greek-style yoghurt masquerading as the real deal. Greek-style yoghurts are often made by adding thickeners or cream to replicate the texture of strained yoghurt, rather than using the authentic straining process. Check the labels and buy what you can afford. I'm not saying there is anything in particular that makes Greek-style yoghurt bad; I still eat it if I can't find Greek. It's just that authentic Greek is a better choice if you can get it. Typical Greek-style yoghurt has around 4.6g of sugar per 100g. But turn your cart towards the authentic Greek yoghurt, and you'll find only 3.3g per 100g.

Switch your breakfast bowl from Greek-style for a few spoonfuls of Greek yoghurt, and you get an impressive 28% reduction in sugar content – that's a teaspoon of sugar a day. Over the course of a year, that's an amazing 1.4kg drop in sugar. It's important to note this isn't added sugar, this is the naturally occurring sugar from lactose in the milk.

Try these swaps:

SWAPS

Flavoured yoghurts → Plain yoghurt
With berries for antioxidants, fibre, and natural sweetness without the added sugar.

Regular yoghurts → Greek yoghurt
For more protein, less sugar.

Protein for breakfast

I'm sure we all know by now that sugary cereal bowls aren't the best way to start the day. Nutritional wisdom tells us to focus on good protein and fats for breakfast.

Protein doesn't just keep you full, it plays a vital role in maintaining muscle mass, regulating hormones, and even supporting immune function, especially as we age.

This is where yoghurt steps into our shopping trolley. It's my daily go-to breakfast, and if you follow a few simple rules, can be your daily healthy breakfast staple too.

Protein is the building block of our bodies. Authentic Greek yoghurt boasts over double the protein content of Greek-style – 9g per 100g compared to just 4g per 100g. This means in a typical 300g bowl, you'll be getting a whopping 27g of protein versus only 12g in Greek-style. That's an extra 15g of protein a day. With a recent survey suggesting 66% of the UK aren't getting enough protein in their diet,[24] this is an important improvement that also helps to fill you up for longer so you can avoid mid-morning sugary snacks.

While authentic Greek yoghurt can be double the price of Greek-style (depending on where you shop), the health benefits make it a worthy investment in my opinion. With double the protein, you get what you pay for, and you're still paying far less than you'd pay for a protein bar.

The branded varieties at 5% fat tend to have the highest protein content (9g per 100g), so I'd be reaching for those over the supermarket varieties.

Spoilt for choice

The other thing I love about the dairy aisle is the wide variety of choice. You've got yoghurt drinks, yoghurt pouches for kids, yoghurt pots for on-the-go and of course kefir, as well as a range of plant-based and lactose-free options for those with intolerances.

Here's a quick swap guide for your next shop:

SWAPS

Yoghurt drinks → Kefir
For a broader range of probiotics to support gut
health without chemical nasties or extra sugar.

Plant-based yoghurts → Lactose-free yoghurts
For fewer additives.

Kids' yoghurts → Plain yoghurt pots or pouches
For less sugar.

Yoghurt drinks are often marketed as convenient ways to top up your probiotics, but most contain 2.5-3 teaspoons of sugar per drink and just one or two strains of bacteria. Kefir, on the other hand, is a traditional fermented milk drink made with live kefir grains, containing dozens of strains of bacteria and yeasts. This diversity gives kefir a much broader probiotic profile, which many studies suggest is better for supporting gut health and digestion. The taste is tangier than a standard yoghurt drink, but its benefits are far greater, and you can opt for plain versions without the added sugar.

If you're looking for genuine daily gut support, kefir is the clear winner here, and you can now find whole bays of kefir in most stores. Pick a kefir drink or yoghurt depending on your preference – either is great. It's also worth noting that, even though kefir is made from milk, the live cultures ferment most of the lactose, which means kefir is naturally very low in lactose and often easier to digest than milk.

Plant-based vs lactose-free

Plant-based yoghurts have surged in popularity in recent years, fuelled by consumers' growing appetite for more eco-friendly choices. Unfortunately, health is not always factored in. Many non-dairy yoghurt alternatives rely on additives such as gums, starches, stabilisers, and sweeteners to mimic the texture of dairy yoghurt. They are often lower in protein too. The best bet here is to look for the coconut-based yoghurts (made from coconut milk, not merely coconut-flavoured dairy yoghurt). They're not cheap – the more premium brands are often the ones which have cleaned up their act and have fewer additives.

If you shop for plant-based dairy alternatives because you don't tolerate dairy well, lactose-free dairy yoghurts are a good option. These are standard yoghurts which have had the lactose removed by adding an enzyme that eats the lactose – retaining all the protein, fats, and nutrients of the milk. If you're intolerant, lactose-free is often the cleaner choice, with fewer additives and more nutrition than many plant-based alternatives.

Kids' yoghurts vs plain

The kids' yoghurt section is often a sugar trap for parents, with pouches and tubes marketed for lunchboxes containing more sugar than some desserts. For example, Frubes have 9.9g sugar per 100g in their strawberry-flavour yoghurt tubes and Müller Rice have 9.7g sugar per 100g in their tubs. Not exactly a healthy daily staple for kids. Plain yoghurt pots or pouches (if you can find them), by contrast, give you all the protein, calcium, and live cultures without the sugar spike. Giving your kids the benefits of dairy without the hidden nasties is really important and a great snack option anytime.

I know your kids might pester for the red yoghurt box, or the one with a cool cartoon character on it, but this is one area where you have to hold your ground. Even if the pack says 'no added sugar' it may contain big dollops of fruit purée, which is essentially fruit without the fibre, and therefore acts in the same way as sugar in your children's bodies. So, ignore the pester power, give your kids plain yoghurt and add some nuts or berries. They will get used to it.

BUTTER AND CHEESE

For decades, butter was painted as a villain on our tea tables, not because it is infuriatingly unspreadable, but for its supposed artery-clogging risks, and we were all advised to swap to margarine to save our hearts. But nutritional science has come a long way since the low-fat frenzy of the 80s and 90s, and it's time to rewrite the story.

Butter vs margarine: spread the truth

Margarine is a man-made product originally created as a cheap butter substitute. To give it that buttery look and feel, manufacturers chemically alter vegetable oils through a process called hydrogenation. This creates trans fats, the kind of fat linked to inflammation, heart disease, and even cancer. Although trans fats are now mostly banned in the UK, many margarines still contain ultra-processed oils, artificial emulsifiers, preservatives, and colourings. That 'heart-healthy' halo? It's largely marketing spin. Even those claiming to use olive oil or pretending to be butter will have UPF oils and ingredients, so you need to check the labels if it's in a plastic tub.

Butter, on the other hand, is a wholefood made from churned cream and maybe a touch of salt. No additives, no laboratory processing. It's rich in fat-soluble vitamins such as A, D, E, and K2, and contains butyrate, which is a short-chain fatty acid that supports gut health and reduces inflammation. Yes, butter might be high in saturated fat, but recent studies show that moderate saturated fat consumption from wholefoods is not the villain it was previously made out to be.

SWAPS

Margarine → Spreadable butter

Ditch the emulsifiers and processed oils for simple churned cream packed with natural vitamins. Watch the Lurpak spreadable though, at only 64% butter. Kerrygold has naturally softer butter in a tub, which is more spreadable as it is gently churned and is a 100% butter.

Margarine → Butter

Ditch the emulsifiers and processed oils for simple churned cream packed with natural vitamins.

Butter → Grass-fed butter

Better taste, more omega-3s, can be spreadable in ten minutes if you just take it out of the fridge ahead of time.

Cheese, please

The cheese aisle is one of my favourite sections of the supermarket. You'll find such a wide variety of choice and flavours from countries all around the world that this really is a place to feast your eyes and tastebuds.

Contrary to popular belief, the world's greatest cheese lovers are not the French. In fact, the Danes take the crown for topping the global charts[25] of cheese consumption, with the average person eating around 28kg per year. That's more than half a kilo of cheese every week!

To be fair, France does rank high in those charts and is famous for what's called the 'French Paradox', which attempts to explain how the French enjoy some of the lowest rates of heart disease in the developed world despite eating around 27kg of cheese a year per person – plus plenty of butter and also wine.

Cheese has had its fair share of bad PR and is often lumped in with indulgent foods because of its fat content. But scratch the surface, and you'll find a nutrient-dense, protein-packed powerhouse that deserves a regular place on your plate.

THE GOOD

Go for the natural and organic classics such as cheddar, parmesan, feta and brie, which are less likely to be messed with because of their heritage. Cottage cheese is a high-protein option too.

THE BAD

Ultra-processed cheese slices and any kind of 'cheese dunkers', which are bulked out with fillers, stabilisers, and artificial additives.

> **THE HEALTHY**
> Any variety of natural cheese is nutrient-dense and protein-rich.

Cheese is essentially fermented milk, and fermentation is your gut's best friend. Many cheeses also contain probiotics (beneficial bacteria) which help to support digestion, and aid the absorption of key nutrients such as calcium, phosphorus, and vitamin K2. A large scientific review[26] including 54 separate studies has shown that "cheese consumption has neutral to moderate benefits for human health".

Try these simple swaps for your health:

SWAPS

Ultra-processed cheese slices → Real cheddar slices
Swap out fillers and emulsifiers for authentic, full-flavour cheese.

Lunchbox cheese snacks → Cottage cheese pots
Higher protein, fewer additives, and keeps you fuller for longer.

Branded cream cheese → Supermarket own-label cream cheese
The well-known leading brands often contain added gums and carrageenan. Instead, check the label on the supermarket's own brand and you might find it contains just one ingredient – milk.

Some brands even offer pre-packed slices of 'cheese' with ham or chicken, which you stack with crackers. If you look at the sample ingredients list below, it's certainly not the kind of cheese we should be giving to our children on a regular basis. Ingredients:

Cheese (75%), skimmed milk (water, skimmed milk powder), emulsifying salts (sodium citrates, potassium citrates), milk proteins, butter, skimmed milk powder, whey powder (from milk) vitamin D, preservative (sorbic acid), acidity regulator (citric acid), anti-caking agent (sunflower lecithins).

I think cottage cheese needs to get an honourable mention in this chapter. It might not be the trendiest tub in your fridge, but nutritionally, it punches well above its weight. With over 11g of protein per 100g and just 80–100 calories, it's one of the leanest, most efficient ways to boost your daily protein.

It is rich in casein, a slow-digesting protein that helps keep hunger at bay for hours. That makes it an ideal snack, breakfast base, or even a smart evening choice to curb late-night cravings. Sweet or savoury, cottage cheese is versatile, affordable, and easy to build into meals. It's not flashy, but it gets the job done and does it better than most.

Another point worth mentioning is that the international cheese scene also has added benefits for your health. Most of the cheeses are made using traditional methods, and in some cases are sold as raw (unpasteurised). These cheeses – like Italian parmesan, French roquefort, and certain Swiss alpine varieties – contain more of the original enzymes and beneficial bacteria that are otherwise destroyed during pasteurisation and heavy processing.

This contributes not only to their complex flavour but also to potential digestive and probiotic benefits. And before people worry about it being raw, cheese has undergone fermentation, acidification, salting, and ageing, all of which reduce pathogens and make it safe to eat.

EGGS

Fried, scrambled, poached, boiled, it doesn't really matter. Eggs are – or should be – a versatile staple on almost everybody's weekly shopping list, but I really don't think they get the credit they deserve.

When it comes to buying eggs, it can be tricky to know which box to pull off the supermarket shelf. The labels, packet health claims and prices vary considerably, but they all taste the same – or do they?

The truth is, not all eggs are created equal, and you can often see the difference the moment you crack an egg into a pan. Cheap, intensively farmed eggs tend to have thin, watery whites and pale yolks, which indicates that the hens have been fed a basic, grain-heavy diet and they've had very little outdoor access. By contrast, a good egg will have a rich, golden yolk surrounded by a firm, gelatinous white. These are clear signs that the egg is fresh and the hens have had the chance to roam outdoors and eat a more varied, natural diet.

Proper quality eggs don't just look better on your plate, they're usually higher in nutrients too.

THE GOOD
Organic or high-welfare free-range eggs: hens get outdoor access and natural feed, resulting in richer yolks and higher omega-3s.

> **THE BAD**
> Intensively farmed caged/barn eggs: cheaper, but hens live in crowded conditions, and the eggs often have lower levels of nutrients.
>
> **THE HEALTHY**
> Free-range eggs: nature's multivitamin, with protein, vitamins A, D, E, B12, choline, lutein, and zeaxanthin.

Eggs truly are nature's multivitamin. Each egg is packed with essential nutrients that our bodies need to function optimally. Price does usually reflect quality in this aisle, but that doesn't mean you always have to buy the most expensive box. A simple upgrade from caged eggs to free-range already improves both welfare and nutrition, as free-range hens have more outside space to roam, with more vitamin D and omega-3s in the yolk. From there, organic is the gold standard: fewer hens per square metre, guaranteed outdoor access, and higher-quality feed, which all translate to richer yolks and better nutrition. A good rule of thumb:

- **On a budget:** always choose at least free-range.
- **Mid-range:** opt for free-range organic if available.
- **Top tier:** look for local farm eggs where the supply chain is shorter, meaning fresher, more nutrient-dense eggs.

Eggs can be one of the most intensely farmed foods in the UK, so it is worth investing in better quality eggs if you can.

SWAPS

Battery eggs → Barn eggs
13–16 birds per square metre and no outdoor access.

Barn eggs → Free-range
9 birds per square metre and guaranteed outdoor access.

Free range → Organic
6 birds per square metre and daily outdoor access for at least one-third of their life.

Organic → Local farm eggs
Fewer food miles and supports your local community directly.[27]

There's a huge difference in nutrition based on the amount of time the chicken spends outdoors. One study shows that the vitamin D3 content of egg yolk was almost four times higher in the chicken groups that were exposed to sunlight.[28] So, it is worth at least making the switch to free-range for your own health, if not for the chicken's quality of life.

Some egg boxes will proudly shout about the golden yolks inside the eggs. These 'enriched' eggs can vary massively in price, and it can be confusing to decide with all the new claims shouting at you from the shelves. One thing is clear: the more nutrition packed in, the better, so enriched eggs can be a good idea, but the golden yolk promises have been overblown. In nature, a darker/brighter yolk means more nutrition. In the poultry world, the chances are these hens are being fed paprika (which is red) and marigold extracts (which are bright yellow) and the colour is migrating to their egg yolks. Unfortunately, you are probably just paying extra for an Instagram-worthy egg that is no better for your health.

Go large

If you want the most egg for your money, compare the price per 100g. As a rule of thumb, large eggs usually work out cheapest because you're getting more egg without a big jump in price.

Here is a quick check you can do if the shelf label doesn't show it:

price per 100g = pack price ÷ (number of eggs × weight) × 100.

In most shops, large eggs work out cheaper than medium or extra-large.

An egg's superpowers

When you read about nutritional 'superfoods', you might see people talking about blueberries, green powders, and goji berries from the Amazon rainforest. But, in my opinion, the humble egg is one of the most nutritious, affordable, and versatile foods you can find in the supermarket, making it the best superfood of all in my book.

Let's compare eggs to other popular superfoods to highlight just how affordable and nutritious they are:

- **Blueberries:** Famous for their antioxidants, but they typically cost almost three times the price of eggs.
- **Green powders:** These supplements promise a concentrated dose of vitamins and minerals, but they often come with a hefty price tag, some up to 15 times more expensive than your average box of eggs.
- **Protein bars**: Marketed as a convenient protein source, but these bars are expensive and they are ultra-processed foods loaded with artificial sweeteners and additives worth avoiding.

So, let's crack into even more reasons why eggs deserve the number-one spot on your shopping list!

Protein: Each egg contains about 6g of high-quality protein, which is vital for muscle repair, immune function, and overall health. Eat three eggs a day and you'll be adding 18g of protein to your diet – but not just ANY protein. Eggs contain so-called 'complete protein', because unlike many other protein sources, they provide all nine essential amino acids (histidine, isoleucine, leucine, lysine, methionine, phenylalanine, threonine, tryptophan, valine), which are the building blocks of our muscles.

Vitamins and minerals: The average egg contains a huge range of nutrients, including:
- Vitamin A: 270IU
- Vitamin D: 41IU
- Vitamin E: 0.5mg

- Vitamin K: 0.1mcg
- Vitamin B2 (riboflavin): 0.25mg
- Vitamin B5 (pantothenic acid): 0.7mg
- Vitamin B6: 0.1mg
- Vitamin B9 (folate): 24mcg
- Vitamin B12: 0.6mcg
- Calcium: 28mg
- Iron: 0.8mg
- Magnesium: 6mg
- Phosphorus: 99mg
- Potassium: 69mg
- Sodium: 70mg
- Zinc: 0.6mg
- Selenium: 15.4mcg
- Copper: 0.025mg
- Manganese: 0.02mg

(based on a medium egg)

These nutrients support everything from vision and bone health to brain function and metabolism and are a great addition to your everyday diet.

Antioxidants: These are compounds that protect the body's cells from damage. Egg yolks contain powerful antioxidants like lutein and zeaxanthin, which are crucial for eye health – but they are also packed with choline, one of the most essential antioxidants, which particularly supports the brain, nervous system, liver, and cell function. Two eggs a day provide 50% of your required choline intake.

So, when looking at the price per kg, it's easy to see what good value eggs are, being 10x cheaper than a typical protein bar per kg. And with the added nutrient profile you get from the amino acids, vitamins and choline, they are, in my opinion, one of the best supermarket superfoods.

Debunking the cholesterol myth

For years, eggs got a bad rap due to their cholesterol content. But thanks to advancements in nutritional science, we now know that the cholesterol in eggs doesn't significantly impact blood cholesterol levels for most people.[29] In fact, studies have shown that eating eggs can actually improve your HDL (good) cholesterol while maintaining the healthy HDL to LDL (bad) cholesterol ratio. So, if you've been avoiding eggs for this reason, it's time to bring them back to the table.

In a world of fad diets and trendy new health crazes, eggs are a classic, affordable, nutrient-dense staple that deserve a place in everybody's trolley.

MEAT AND FISH

Walk down the chilled meat aisle and you might initially think the good, bad and healthy choices are easy to spot. But in reality, the good stuff is harder to find. Fifty or so years ago, fatty cuts of meat were prized because they were thought to carry the most flavour and energy. Lean cuts like rump were often considered less satisfying. But today, we are all over the 5%-fat (i.e. low-fat) mince and the expensive lean cuts in a bid to protect our health, thanks to the common belief that saturated fat – found in meat, cheese and butter – is something to be avoided.

Yet, the latest science suggests that saturated fat and cholesterol may not be as harmful as researchers once thought they were. A 2020 review[30] that investigated several studies on saturated fat and heart disease found that the association between the two appears to be very weak.[31]

You might be surprised to learn that fatty meat also stores more nutrients than lean. Vitamins like A, D, E, and K are fat-soluble and stored in animal fat. So, that delicious lean fillet steak may actually contain fewer nutrients than the cheaper, fattier piece of steak.

THE GOOD
Grass-fed and/or organic fattier meats such
as 20%-fat mince or ribeye steak.

All hail beef mince

With saturated fat no longer a worry, let's turn to the healthiest option for you and your wallet: move over fillet steak, there is a new cut in town.

Minced beef has plenty of fat-soluble vitamins and nutrients – but that's not all. A good mince will also contain fragments of tendons, ligaments and connective tissue, which are a fantastic natural source of collagen.

Collagen is a protein full of amino acids that supports the structure of your skin, hair, and nails. It also plays a vital role in maintaining the integrity of your joints and connective tissues. By choosing minced beef with 20% fat, you're getting a broader nutritional profile, including around 15g of collagen, which you might well pay a lot of money for if it was a supplement. Most supplements deliver about 5g of collagen.

Not only does minced beef save you money, but it also provides a versatile base for countless dishes: burgers, meatballs, bolognese, tacos…the possibilities are endless. It's the affordable option that gives you the healthiest upside, with all the added fat-soluble vitamins, omega-3s and collagen.

SWAPS

Fillet steak → Ribeye steak
Ribeye is a delicious treat with added fat,
which offers more fat-soluble vitamins for
30% less of your hard-earned money.

Ribeye steak → Sirloin steak
Sirloin is one of the most economical ways
to eat steak and that nice rind of fat
gives you added nutrition.

Sirloin steak → 5%-fat minced beef
Premium mince, but less than half the price of your
average steak, making it a great affordable option.
Chose the lower-fat content only if you're aiming
to reduce calories.

5%-fat mince → 20%-fat minced beef
20%-fat mince offers higher nutrition
for a lower price.

Intensively farmed beef → Grass-fed beef
Six times more omega-3s and a cleaner nutrient profile.
Although all unprocessed meat is healthy, you score
extra health points if you're picky about the way your
animals are reared. Typically, cows reared on grass
will produce beef that is 6x higher in Omega-3
fatty acids, which are beneficial for heart and brain
health, than industrially farmed cattle (called 'feedlot'
cattle in the US) which are usually fed on grain.

Boneless cuts → On-the-bone cuts
Better value and added minerals from bones/broth.

Bird is the word

The most popular meat in the UK is chicken – it accounts for almost half of all meat consumed daily. It might be a go-to staple, but in my opinion, most of us are buying and eating it wrong. If you're putting chicken breasts or boneless thighs in your shopping basket each week, you're probably missing out on both nutrition and money savings.

Most people have a long-standing preference for chicken breast because it's lean, low in fat and easy to handle. But it's the same story as beef: fat is NOT the enemy! There's a lot of goodness stored in the parts we usually discard, such as the skin, bones, and darker meat cuts such as chicken thighs and legs, which are richer in essential nutrients such as collagen, zinc, iron, and fat-soluble vitamins A and K2.

THE GOOD
Whole organic chicken gives you more meals, better nutrient density, and it is cheaper gram-for-gram.

THE BAD
Chicken kievs, nuggets, deep-fried. You name it, anything in this processed category is heavily laden with batter, bread and oils. Usually anywhere from 30-40%.

THE HEALTHY
If you tend to eat pre-prepared chicken, start cooking from scratch. Any unprocessed chicken is a good protein source, and you'll be minimising the chemical additives that are so bad for your health.

You might reel at the idea of splashing out on an organic whole chicken, but when you do the 'bird maths', it works out not only cheaper per kilogram than buying individual non-organic chicken parts, but it also gives you a broader nutritional profile. Whenever I buy chicken, I always aim to roast the whole bird with the idea that it will feed the family for days. We have that roast chicken on the first night, followed by leftover legs and thighs the next day, and then we use the bones to make a nourishing broth which forms the basis of soup or risotto on the third day. One bird, three meals, which give you the full nutrition complex of the bird without breaking the bank.

In fact, swapping a weekly 500g pack of chicken breasts for one whole organic chicken can triple the amount of food you are getting for the same price and feed you better quality food for days longer.

Try these swaps:

SWAPS

Chicken breast → Bone-in thighs or legs
More flavour, more nutrients and more collagen.

Non-organic → Organic
Fewer antibiotics, better omega-3s, tastier meat.

Lean meat → Chicken livers
One of the most nutrient-dense foods in the world.

A note on quality: choose organic chicken wherever possible. Poultry is one of the most intensively farmed animals, and quality matters hugely. Organic chickens are raised with better feed, fewer antibiotics, and in more humane conditions with more space to roam, which results in tastier, more nutrient-dense meat.

If you've got the stomach for it, there is one cut of chicken that is also super-affordable and is officially one of the most nutrient-dense foods in the world. Please put your hands together for chicken livers – one of the most economical protein and nutrient sources out there. At the time of writing, they cost about the same as chicken thighs on the bone, but they pack a much more powerful nutrient punch.

Chicken livers should really be touted as a superfood due to their high nutrient density. They are an exceptional source of vitamin A, which is crucial for vision, immune function, and skin health. They also boast high levels of B vitamins, particularly B12, which is vital for brain health and energy production. Additionally, chicken livers are rich in folate and iron. The difference is stark.

While you might be hesitant about the taste or texture of chicken livers, they are incredibly versatile and can be prepared in ways that make them more palatable, from pâtés to sautéed dishes with onions. My go-to is simple: fry them quickly with onions, mushrooms and a spicy sauce.

Bangers, bacon and burgers

Now let's turn to the classic staples of the British fry-up or BBQ, as they sit in a very different category from fresh cuts of meat. Bacon, sausages and most burgers on the supermarket shelf are processed meats, which means they have been salted, cured, smoked, or bulked out with fillers and preservatives to extend shelf life and enhance flavour.

The problem is that those processes often come with a health cost. Nitrites, commonly used in bacon and sausages, are linked to increased risk of colorectal cancer, while added starches, seed oils and fillers dilute the nutrient profile of the actual meat.[32] Many budget sausages and burgers contain less than 70% meat, topped up with breadcrumbs, rusk, vegetable oils and flavour enhancers – so you're not getting the nutritional benefits you think you are. Regular consumption of processed meats has been associated with higher rates of disease. But don't worry, I love a good burger and, as always, there are ways to do in a healthier form.

Because not all sausages and burgers are equal. If you're selective, there are healthier swaps that let you enjoy these foods in moderation without the worst downsides. Look for options with at least 90-95% meat content, ideally free from nitrites. Many butchers now offer clean label sausages made from just meat, herbs and spices. For burgers, it's often better value and healthier to buy some good quality mince and shape your own patties – it only takes a few minutes to make burgers at home.

THE GOOD
Make your own burgers or buy minimally processed
sausages from a butcher or the store that are nitrite-free.

THE BAD
Mass-produced sausages, burgers and bacon loaded
with fillers, nitrites, vegetable oils and flavourings.
Some sausages are as low as 42% pork.

THE HEALTHY
High-meat content sausages and burgers (90%+)
and ideally nitrite-free.

The dish on fish

Far too many of us walk right past the fresh fish aisle in
the supermarket, or perhaps stop to pick up a nice, safe
and familiar piece of boneless salmon or cod fillet. But if
you're keen to maximise your nutrition, it's a good idea
to consider buying wild-caught fish – and you might just
want to head over to the freezer section for that.

THE GOOD
Wild fish such as salmon, sea bass, mackerel,
sardines, which provide a rich source of omega-3s.

THE BAD
Processed, breaded or battered fish, and farmed fish
fed on processed pellets, often with lower nutrients
and potential residues.

Farmed fish, especially salmon, has become a supermarket staple. It's easy, convenient, and often cheaper per portion to buy. But did you know that farmed salmon is often fed pellets with added synthetic colourants to turn the flesh that classic orange-pink salmon colour? In the wild, the colour comes from krill in their natural diet, but without colourants in their food, farmed salmon would be an unappetising grey colour.

Because they have the freedom to roam and eat their natural diet of plankton, algae, and smaller fish, the flesh from wild fish is much richer in omega-3 fatty acids, vitamin D, selenium, and a powerful antioxidant called astaxanthin. These nutrients are great for brain health, inflammation control, and heart protection. By contrast, farmed fish are typically raised on processed feed, which lowers their nutritional quality and increases harmful chemical residues.

I know wild fish are more expensive; you find yourself paying triple the price in the blink of an eye, making a wild salmon steak more expensive than a quality beef steak. But luckily, there are some clever swaps to help you save your money.

SWAPS

Farmed salmon → Wild salmon
Eat the real deal and boost your nutrition.

Boneless fillets → Whole fish
A whole fish provides not just the fillets, but the skin and bones too, which are rich in collagen, calcium, and other minerals. Use the bones to make a broth and you'll stretch your money further while nourishing your body more deeply.

Fresh → Frozen
The fresh fish on supermarket shelves has often been previously frozen, so you may as well head to the freezer and save yourself some money. When you are freezing fish soon after it is caught, the supply chain is simpler and less expensive, which helps to bring the price down.

Just by swapping your weekly two farmed fresh salmon fillets for wild frozen fillets, you'll save around 25% and increase the quality of your nutrition. That's a win for your wallet and your wellbeing.

Eat the little fishies

One of the concerns you often hear is that, if you eat a lot of fish, you might end up consuming mercury, a heavy metal that accumulates in the flesh of sea creatures as you go up the food chain. When we eat it, mercury can affect the nervous system, and eating too much is particularly risky for children and pregnant women.

Small fish eat plankton, which absorb mercury from water and sediment, and that mercury can build up in their tissues. Smaller oily fish such as sardines, mackerel, and anchovies sit low in the food chain, so they contain far less mercury than larger fish, while still delivering the same omega-3s and nutrients that make fish such a health powerhouse.

But when larger predatory fish such as tuna, sword-fish, and shark eat these smaller fish, the levels of mercury accumulate over time. The bigger the fish and the longer it has lived, the more likely it is to have high mercury levels in its tissues. Try to eat a variety of low-mercury fish, especially if you are pregnant or breastfeeding.

SUPERMARKET FAST FOOD

Let's be honest: we all have days when time is tight, energy is low, and the idea of prepping a proper dinner is laughable. That's real life. With my two kids and 10-hour workdays, I often can't find the time or energy to cook and I can see the temptation of an oven pizza or a microwave ready meal.

The good news? Fast food doesn't have to mean junk food. With a bit of planning and a few simple swaps, you can still eat well without spending hours in the kitchen. When I know I'm going to be short on cooking time, I make sure I've got a couple of these simple healthy meals ready to go.

THE GOOD
Homemade tray bakes are the ultimate fast meal with high-quality nutrition from whatever you have in the fridge.

THE BAD
Microwave meals and frozen pizzas with low nutritional value and limited vegetables.

THE HEALTHY
Stir-fry kits can be just as fast as microwave meals and have tonnes of fresh vegetables for a nutrient fix.

Switch ready meals for meal kits

Microwave meals might seem like an easy option on chaotic evenings, but many are loaded with low-quality ingredients, too much salt, preservatives, and hidden UPF fats to make them shelf-stable and 'tasty'. But they are usually nutritionally poor. A standard microwaveable chicken and bacon pasta bake only contains 11% chicken, for instance, and no vegetables apart from a bit of garlic purée. The best-selling microwave meal in the UK is chicken tikka masala, which often contains only 21% chicken, and again has no vegetables other than tomato purée for the sauce and some onion and garlic for taste.

For a smarter swap, try fresh stir-fry kits. These are widely available in supermarkets now, usually in the fridge section on a combo deal. They come with pre-chopped veg and often a little sauce packet. Just toss the veg into a hot pan with coconut or olive oil, add your choice of protein – chicken, prawns, tofu – and cook for 5-10 minutes. You'll have dinner on the table faster than waiting for a delivery.

Pro tip: make your own sauce. Those little sachets of teriyaki sauce can have up to 24g of sugar, which is wild. An easy stir-fry sauce can be made in minutes with soy sauce, lime juice, garlic and ginger – plus a little honey to balance the flavours if you like.

Switch pizza for pittas

Frozen oven pizzas are classic freezer staples, but they're typically packed with refined carbs, processed meats, and are usually almost entirely devoid of vegetables and therefore woefully lacking in nutrients. A super-easy alternative? Homemade pitta pizzas. Just grab wholemeal pitta breads (one of the supermarkets original non-UPF breads) and top them with passata, a sprinkle of cheese, and whatever veggies you might find lurking in the fridge such as mushrooms or even broccoli, which goes surprisingly well on a pizza. Pop them in a hot oven for about eight minutes until the cheese is melted and golden and your dinner is ready to be served. It's all the joy of pizza night, with more fibre, less grease, and you still get to eat it with your hands. If you want to make the meal more well-rounded, increase the protein by adding mozzarella and some unprocessed meat, or crack an egg on top.

Pimp up your burger and chips

Sometimes you just want a burger and chips. There's no shame in that. We are all human. But a drive-thru burger meal can hit your health hard because it is loaded with processed buns, sugary sauces and fries dunked in old oil. A fast-food burger bun might have up to 17 ingredients —and the cheese slice is often only 60% cheese. Even if you only eat like this occasionally, it's still not a great way to eat and fuel your body. The good news? You can make an even tastier version at home in under 30 minutes, and it's way better for you.

Start with beef mince – the fattier the better if you

like your burger juicy. Season it with salt, pepper, maybe a little garlic powder or smoked paprika, and shape into patties. No fillers required. Sear them in a hot pan and add a slice of real cheese on top at the end. Serve on their own or even wrapped in crisp lettuce leaves, with some fresh tomato, onion, pickles, and a little ketchup.

For your chips, skip the deep fat fryer. Instead, slice up potatoes (or sweet potatoes), toss with olive oil, salt and pepper, then roast at 220°C for about 25 minutes, turning once. It's even quicker if you have an air fryer. Your chips will come out crispy on the edges and you avoid the dodgy fats that come with fast-food fries.

It's real food, real flavour, and you still get to enjoy burger night with no regrets.

SWAPS

Microwave ready meals → Stir-fry kits
Ready in under 10 minutes, no chopping required and a deliciously healthy alternative to ready meals, which have limited nutrition.

Frozen pizza → Homemade pitta pizza
Fast and so easy to make that the kids can join in.

Fast-food burger → Homemade burger
None of the deep-fried nonsense, 100% of the same pleasure.

Traybake magic

Here's one of my absolute go-to solutions for those 'too tired to think' nights. Roughly chop whatever veggies you have – things like peppers, courgettes, onions, cherry tomatoes and aubergines work brilliantly – and toss them on a baking tray with olive oil, garlic salt and pepper. Nestle in a few chicken thighs. Bake at 200°C for about 35 minutes. In the last 5 mins, crumble over some feta.

It's unbelievably simple, hands-off, and the oven does all the work. The beauty of this dish is that it literally doesn't matter what you have in the fridge – just grab whatever you can find, chuck it in the oven and out comes a delicious and tasty meal. Convenience doesn't have to mean compromise, and sometimes health isn't about being perfect, it's just about making the choice a little bit easier and better.

PASTA, RICE AND GRAINS

Carbs have had a rough decade. From keto to paleo to low-carb everything, we've been told to treat grains like the nutritional villain. But don't just stroll right past the aisle with all the different pastas, rice and grain products, because the discussion is way more nuanced. More detailed advice should help you navigate this aisle and make a few healthy choices that might surprise you.

Until the 19th century, almost all grains eaten around the world were whole, milled slowly on stone wheels and often fermented, sprouted, or soaked before cooking. The invention of industrial roller mills in the late 1800s changed that. For the first time, the bran and germ could be stripped away cheaply, leaving behind fluffy white flour with a long shelf life but little nutritional value. This innovation fuelled everything from white bread to instant noodles, but it also marked the beginning of refined carbs dominating the modern diet. Here's the truth: grains alone aren't the problem – it's how we ultra-process them and the amount we consume that causes the issue.

I get it, they're one of the cheapest ways to feed a family and can provide an easy and fast addition to any meal. But notice the key word: addition. Most people tend to take grains as the base of any meal: a big pile of rice or pasta then a little bit of whatever you choose to put with it. But this is the wrong way around. Many grains are high in energy, but very low in micronutrients. So, we should be thinking of flipping our plate choices around and asking:

1) What healthy meat or vegetables will lead this meal?
2) How can I incorporate some healthy fats into this?
3) What grains can complement this meal, or do I need to add grains to this at all?

Most of the meals I cook at home simply focus on meat and vegetables with olive oil. There is nothing more complicated to eating healthily than sticking to meat and vegetables. But I appreciate that carbs and grains are super-delicious, high in energy and can be part of a healthy meal, so let's get into the nitty-gritty of healthy grains.

THE GOOD
Properly prepared grains (soaked, sprouted, fermented, or cooled/reheated). These methods reduce anti-nutrients, lower glycaemic impact, and boost gut health.

THE BAD
Refined grains such as white bread, white rice, instant noodles and boxed cereals, because they are nutrient-poor, and the body digests them super-fast, triggering a spike in blood sugar levels.

THE HEALTHY
Whole grains such as brown rice, oats, spelt, rye, and quinoa, which retain their fibre, vitamins, minerals, and healthy fats.

Good grains vs empty grains

Not all grains are created equal. *Whole* grains contain the bran, germ and endosperm, which is where the goodness hides – all the fibre, healthy fats, and nutrients. *Refined* grains, on the other hand, such as white bread, white pasta, and instant noodles, are stripped of the bran and germ, which means they lose most of the nutrients and fibre.

Refined grains get digested fast, spike blood sugar, and leave you hungry again quickly. Whole grains are digested more slowly, fuelling your gut microbiome, and keeping you feeling fuller for longer.

Who doesn't love pasta?

Pasta has become a staple in almost everyone's kitchen and our love affair with Italian pasta shows no signs of slowing. Whether it's lasagne, spaghetti or macaroni cheese that gets your mouth watering, in the UK we eat roughly 4kg of pasta a year – about a bowl a week.

The many different shapes – from rice-like orzo, bowtie farfalle, shell-like conchiglie, twisted fusilli or hollow rigatoni – are cleverly designed to optimise whatever sauce is being served. For example, long, thin strands like spaghetti suit light, oily sauces, while ridged, or hollow shapes are designed to hold thicker sauces packed with added ingredients.

Although a big plate of pasta is often dismissed as carbohydrate-heavy comfort food, I think it plays a very useful role in a healthy diet. There is so much complexity and art that goes into crafting the different shapes, and

I'll show you how making one simple swap can transform your pasta into a protein and fibre-packed meal.

The first thing to say is that it's worth paying a little extra for a good-quality brand. The lowest-cost pasta is usually made from refined wheat flour, which is stripped of the bran and wheat germ, meaning it is low in protein, fibre and other nutrients. Cheap pasta might deliver about 5-6g of protein per 100g, which adds up to 10-12g if you eat a big bowlful.

But a proper Italian branded pasta is made using course semolina flour extracted from grinding top-quality durum wheat. Italian pasta makers have to adhere to strict government standards, which dictate how their pasta is made. They must select the best durum wheat in terms of gluten quality, healthiness and protein content, as well as giving it extended drying time, which allows for a more relaxed gluten structure that makes proper Italian pasta easier to digest.

Wholewheat pasta is another great swap as it retains the bran and germ of the wheat kernel, making it higher in both fibre and micronutrients compared to refined pasta. For wholewheat you are getting 7.6g of fibre per 100g or 25% of your daily intake. That's nearly triple what you'd get from standard white pasta. The extra fibre slows digestion, improves satiety, supports gut health, and helps stabilise blood sugar levels.

THE GOOD

Traditional Italian durum wheat pasta: slightly higher protein and better texture thanks to semolina. Organic if you can afford it.

THE BAD

Refined white supermarket pasta: lowest in protein (5–6g/100g) and fibre, turning this into a fast-digesting carbohydrate likely to spike blood sugar levels.

THE HEALTHY

Wholewheat or legume-based pasta (made from lentil or chickpea flour): higher in fibre and protein to support gut health, slow glucose release, and keep you fuller for longer.

High-protein pasta

Pasta made from legumes such as lentils or chickpeas is gaining popularity because, although not classically Italian, the legume content means you get much more protein. It averages out at about 12-13 grams per 100g, which means a 200g plate of legume pasta delivers 24-26g of protein before you add any meat or protein into the sauce!

But this kind of pasta has other important health benefits too. It boasts 25%-50% more fibre than standard pasta, which means it helps keep you fuller for longer, and it is gluten-free.

Fibre is a key component of a heathy diet and most of us aren't getting enough. In fact Public Health England data estimates only 9% of people in the UK are getting the recommended 30g of fibre in their diet each day. This is what makes lentil pasta a gamechanger. A generous 200g serving delivers 6.4g of fibre per plate, which is 21% of your daily intake. Fibre will also help slow your body's metabolism of the sugars in the carbohydrate, which makes high-fibre pasta a useful switch if you want to keep your blood sugar levels under control.

Major supermarkets are catching onto the 'pack protein into everything' health wave, and are now offering a variety of higher-protein pastas with more of the higher protein duram wheat (Tesco High Protein Penne, for instance, is 8.8% protein and 3.2% fibre).

SWAPS

White pasta → Wholewheat pasta
Same price but double the fibre.

Supermarket basics pasta → Branded Italian pasta
Pay a little more for semolina quality, higher protein content and longer-lasting energy.

White pasta → Lentil or chickpea pasta
Double the protein, gluten-free, and higher fibre (though more expensive).

Legume pasta can start to look quite pricey — roughly double the price of normal branded pasta — and that's why I recommend basing your pasta choices on your personal priorities, whether that's budget or health. I sometimes choose branded Italian pasta over lentil pasta for my family because we tolerate gluten well.

But if you can afford to eat lentil or chickpea pasta, it's

a good investment in your health. You'd need to pay out an extra pound or two a week – over £90 a year (based on eating one pack a week) – but in return you get the triple health benefits of more protein, more fibre and it's gluten free. If budgets are tight and fibre is your focus, simply making the switch to wholewheat pasta is the best option for you. You will notice feeling fuller for longer with each plate and the fibre will also support better gut health over time.

Take your pick… but it is definitely time to upgrade your pasta.

Even with the healthiest pasta bubbling away on your hob, it can tip over into a carb-heavy meal if portions get too large. A restaurant portion, for instance, can easily hit 300g or the equivalent of four or five slices of white bread. When you're cooking pasta at home, aim for 80-100g dried pasta per person, and balance your plate properly with added meat and plenty of vegetables and, of course, cheese for the good fats.

Pasta works best as part of a balanced meal, and not the main event. With smarter choices like wholewheat, branded Italian or legumes, and right-sized portions with added meat and vegetables, you get the comfort of pasta without the carb crash.

Rice is nice

Rice deserves a mention here because it's at the heart of so many meals and there are some handy ways to level up your rice game. Basmati rice is the standout if you prefer white rice. Thanks to its naturally lower glycaemic index, it gives a slower and steadier release of energy compared to most other white varieties, which means fewer spikes in your blood sugar. Brown rice, on the other hand, keeps the grain's bran and germ intact, which means more fibre. It takes a little longer to cook and can be harder to digest unless you soak it, but nutritionally speaking, it's a clear upgrade.

The only caveat is that rice plants are very absorbent and naturally accumulate a little arsenic from soil and water, most of which is stored in the bran. That means brown rice can sometimes carry more arsenic than white rice, which has the bran stripped away. So, while brown rice is usually the healthier choice, eating a mix of grains and not relying on brown rice every day is the smart move. But the starting point is:

SWAPS

White rice → Brown basmati
For more fibre and steadier energy release.

White rice → Wild rice
For more antioxidants, fewer calories and less carbs.

If you want to step things up another level, wild rice is the hidden gem of the rice family. Technically a grass, not a true rice, it's higher in protein, fibre, and antioxidants than both white and brown rice. It has a nutty, earthy flavour and chewy texture that makes any dish more satisfying. It's also less likely to carry high arsenic levels, making it a brilliant addition to your weekly rotation.

But rice isn't the only grain worth considering. There are plenty of alternatives making their way onto our shelves. Quinoa has shot to fame as a supergrain and its secret is it's technically a seed, which makes it rich in fibre, minerals, and all nine essential amino acids. A grain that is a complete protein source.

Buckwheat is another great option; it brings an earthy flavour and is packed with fibre and with antioxidants like rutin that support circulation and heart health. Pearl barley is another classic that's being rediscovered, rich in beta-glucans – a type of soluble fibre that helps to keep blood sugar levels in check – and with a lovely chewy texture that makes meals more satisfying. Below is a handy table ranking the grains based on protein and fibre content, which will help you feel fuller and create a more balanced meal.

Healthy grains leaderboard

Rank	Grain	Protein (g/100 g)	Fibre (g/100 g)
1	Quinoa	4.4	2.8
2	Brown basmati	4.9	1.6
3	Buckwheat	3.4	2.7
4	Pearl barley	2.2	3.8
5	Brown rice (long-grain)	2.7	1.6
6	White basmati	2.7	0.4
7	White rice (long-grain)	2.7	0.4

Source: myfooddata.com & nutritionvalue.org [33-39]

The point here is that you don't have to stick with the same old white rice as the base of every meal. If you get creative and mix it up but working your way up the rankings, you will find another type of rice or grain that will help you on your health journey. Choose what you like best but aim for more protein and fibre and you will be on the right path.

One final point to mention is all those plastic pouches of pre-cooked rice. Microplastics are a thing best avoided and, when you microwave those pouches, they may leach microplastics into your food. If you buy them, please always heat in a pan. Another consideration is that these pouches are commonly pasteurised in the factory to make them shelf-stable. This is done by heating the sealed pouches in hot water, maintaining the internal temperature at levels that kill bacteria. Great for killing bacteria, not so great for microplastics potentially leaching into your food. That's why I always try and cook my rice at home if I can. It's far cheaper too.

Nudge up the health of your carbohydrates

Now, it's not just the type of grain but also how, when and why you are eating them that can make a difference to the overall health profile of your carbohydrates:

1. Strategic timing

The key is when and why you're eating them. If you're about to go for a run, hit the gym, or you have a physically demanding day ahead, carbohydrates can be the perfect energy source. They help top up muscle glycogen and give you fuel for performance. But if you're just about to plonk yourself at a desk for the next eight hours, that carb load isn't needed. In that context, a big bowl of porridge or a stack of white toast for breakfast mainly gives you a glucose surge, followed by insulin doing its job to clear your blood sugar, and then the classic mid-morning slump. This is why so many people reach for snacks a couple of hours after a carb-heavy meal. The carbs weren't wrong, the timing was. It's about being strategic:

SWAPS

A big carb meal on a desk or TV day → Big up the fibrous veggies, protein or fats instead of carbs.

A no-carb meal before an active day → A big carb meal to fuel your body for action.

---

2. Soak, batch cook, reheat

By preparing them properly, you not only make your carbohydrates more nutritious but also easier on your digestion. Grains naturally come with a compound called phytic acid, which is often dubbed an anti-nutrient. Phytic acid binds to minerals such as iron, zinc, and magnesium, reducing how much your gut can absorb. But if you soak grains in warm water (with a splash of lemon juice or apple cider vinegar) for several hours, you can kickstart the breakdown of phytic acid, freeing up these minerals for absorption. If I am having rice in the evening, I will always try and remember to soak the rice at least a few hours before cooking. It doesn't always happen but it's always worth trying.

SWAPS

Dry grains → Soaked or sprouted grains
Soaking breaks down phytic acid, boosts mineral absorption, and makes digestion easier.

Interestingly, cooling and reheating grains transforms some of their digestible starches into resistant starch, a type of carbohydrate that resists digestion in the small intestine and instead feeds your good gut bacteria in the colon. This process lowers the glycaemic impact of grains, leading to smaller blood sugar spikes. So that leftover cold rice or reheated oats might actually be metabolically friendlier than freshly cooked.

SWAPS

Freshly cooked grains → Cooled grains
More resistant starch, lower blood sugar spikes, better for gut health.

---

3. Try fermentation

One of the best ways to enjoy grains? Ferment them. Traditional cultures soaked, sprouted, or fermented grains such as tempeh in Indonesia (fermented soy) or dosa in South India (made from fermented rice and lentils). Sourdough bread isn't just a hipster trend. The long fermentation process to create the air-filled loaf also has a few brilliant health implications:

- **Breaks down gluten and phytic acid:** This makes sourdough easier to digest for many people who are sensitive to gluten (though it is still not safe for coeliacs).
- **Lowers glycaemic index:** Sourdough bread tends to raise blood sugar more slowly than standard white bread.
- **Feeds your gut:** The organic acids produced in the fermentation process become a little prebiotic treat for your gut bacteria.

SWAPS

White toast → Sourdough or rye
Lower GI, easier to digest, and prebiotic benefits.

Carbs and grains aren't the enemy. It's the refined, fast-digesting, eaten-at-the-wrong-time, processed versions that let us down. With some thoughtful preparation and smarter pairing, grains can absolutely be part of a healthy, satisfying diet. Just keep them in context, a supporting role to the main event, meat and vegetables.

BREAKFAST CEREALS

I get it. Trying to get the family ready and out of the door each morning can be like a military operation. A bowl of cereal can be the easiest option when you just need something the kids will eat without making a fuss.

Greek yoghurt is my go-to way to start the day – and scrambled eggs is another breakfast of champions – but if you just can't get the kids to change from cereal, or the hustle of morning routines is too much, let's crunch through the facts and find out how to make your cereal pack a healthier punch.

In any supermarket, the cereal section is likely to be a double-sided mega-aisle of exciting-looking boxes emblazoned with cartoon characters, free toys inside the box, and splashed with 'heart healthy!' and 'high in fibre!' health claims. But there's no getting away from the fact that a cereal breakfast misses a fundamental trick: we need protein and good fats for our first meal of the day, to really fill us up and get us going. Cereal is a good source of neither. In fact, it successfully delivers a sugar and carbohydrate-heavy mini-meal, which causes your blood sugar to spike and pretty much guarantees you will be feeling hungry way before lunch time.

Take a glance at any of the nutrition labels and you'll see the problem. Some popular brands contain 35% sugar or up to 12g per 30g serving. To put that in perspective, that's more sugar gram for gram than some cakes, and it's already half of the daily recommended sugar intake for children! Next time you watch your child digging in, just think: they're eating the equivalent of a spoonful of cereal, and then a spoonful of sugar, then another spoonful of cereal before another full spoonful of sugar. It is most definitely not a good way to start your day.

That 12g of sugar? That's if you carefully weigh yourself a 30g portion. Try it one day. It's TINY! Most people eat double that. According to research, the average bowl of cereal weighs more like 73g than 30g. That means your child could be having their entire daily sugar quota for breakfast before school. And we wonder why they struggle to sit still.

THE GOOD

Greek yoghurt, porridge, eggs are the way to start your day.

THE BAD

Sugar bombs like Frosties (37% sugar) and Crunchy Nut (35%). A single bowl can deliver a child's full daily sugar allowance before school.

THE HEALTHY

Low-sugar, high-fibre cereals such as Weetabix (4.2% sugar, 10% fibre) or All-Bran, which release energy slowly to keep you feeling fuller for longer. Protein cereals can also make for a filling option.

The science backs this up quite conclusively. A 2007 study[33] compared the effects of different breakfasts cereals on children's cognitive performance, by looking at the glycaemic index (or GI) of different cereals. All foods can be given a GI score, which indicates whether they raise blood sugar levels quickly or slowly. You'd expect a glucose spike after eating a high-GI food and a more sustained glucose curve after eating a low-GI food. The study revealed that a low-GI cereal, such as All-Bran, significantly reduced the decline in attention and memory over the morning compared to a high-GI cereal like Frosties. This is a really important point, because even if you're not too fussed about what your children eat, you'll probably care deeply about their performance in school. You want to them to be able to focus, right?

This study also confirms my theory that you don't have to abandon the foods you love and take the expensive high ground. There are always better options available without having to totally change your habits if you don't want to.

So, let's get into the healthier swaps that can make your choices a little healthier.

The key to a healthier cereal bowl is to ensure minimal sugar and maximum fibre, which helps slow down the release of the sugars. So, this is where options like Weetabix come to the forefront as a better option at just 4.2% sugar and 10% fibre.

SWAPS

Crunchy Nut (35% sugar) → Cheerios (17% sugar)
Cut sugar by 50% without losing crunch.

Frosties (37% sugar) → Coco Pops (17% sugar)
Halve sugar while enjoying a chocolatey taste.

Cheerio's (17% sugar) → Cornflakes (8% sugar) Another 50% drop for an easy win. Try not to add your own sugar – but even if you do add a small teaspoon of honey, it would still contain 25% less sugar than Cheerios.

Coco Pops (17% sugar) → Weetabix (4.2%)
Add fibre, slash sugar by 75% and aim to sweeten naturally with berries.

Other notable mentions with lower sugar include:
→ **Shreddies (12.5%)**
→ **Rice Krispies (7.9%)**
→ **Bitesize Shredded Wheat (0.7%)**

However, if you're looking for the best breakfast for you or your kids, it may be time to break up with cereal altogether and consider these alternatives. They all have a far lower GI through higher protein and good fat content.

Greek yoghurt: High in protein and packed with probiotics, Greek yoghurt is my breakfast go-to. Top it with some fresh berries and a sprinkle of nuts or seeds for a fibre and antioxidant boost.

Porridge: Oats are a great breakfast staple, offering a good dose of fibre – but context matters. It's great before a run or the gym, but if you are just sitting at your desk all day it will spike your blood sugar. However, if you add toppings like peanut butter, berries, chia seeds or protein powder, it creates a filling breakfast that will keep your blood sugar levels steadier.

Eggs: Boiled, poached, or scrambled, eggs are a protein-rich option that can keep you fuelled till lunch. Pair them with sourdough toast for a very well-rounded breakfast.

Now, I know what you're thinking... cereal is cheap. If we take the average cereal bowl at 70-75g, with about 250ml of milk, over a year that could be costing you a few hundred pounds for the privilege of an estimated 9-10kg of sugar per year.

However, a typical medium free-range egg is often every bit as affordable as your morning cereal – with far better nutrition. Three eggs on a slice of sourdough comes to roughly the same annual cost: a few hundred pounds a year. So, you can swap over 18g of sugar every morning for over 18g of protein (and all the health benefits that prompts) for only a small weekly difference in cost. Think of it as a health investment.

Switching to these alternatives can drastically cut down your sugar intake and increase your energy levels. A healthy breakfast doesn't just fuel your body; it sets the tone for your entire day. Choose wisely and eat well!

OIL

If there's one item in your kitchen that touches almost every meal you cook, it's oil. Whether you're roasting vegetables, frying an egg, or dressing a salad, oil is going to be involved. For centuries, the Mediterranean diet has been lauded as one of the healthiest in the world and a big part of that comes down to olive oil. In fact, back in the 1960s the Greeks were getting up to 40% of their calories from olive oil – yet they had some of the lowest rates of heart disease of any nation in the world.

Unfortunately, these days cheap refined seed oils such as sunflower and rapeseed oil dominate our diets. The difference isn't just tradition; it's nutrition, and after decades of listening to bad information, most people are getting this daily staple wrong.

Let's start with the basics. Fat isn't the enemy, it's essential. Your body needs fat to absorb vitamins A, D, E and K, build hormones, support brain health, and keep your skin glowing.

But the type of fat you eat matters.

THE GOOD

Extra virgin olive oil (EVOO) is the gold standard. It is rich in polyphenols, stable when heated, and protective against inflammation and heart disease.

> **THE BAD**
> Refined seed oils such as sunflower, rapeseed
> and 'vegetable oil' blends, which are highly processed,
> omega-6 heavy, and stripped of nutrients.
>
> **THE HEALTHY**
> Olive oil, and natural oils like avocado oil, coconut oil,
> and ghee (clarified butter often used in Indian cuisine),
> which retain antioxidants, vitamins, and healthy fats.

One of the biggest myths about oils is that extra virgin olive oil isn't safe for cooking because of its low smoke point. The truth is that EVOO is remarkably stable under heat, thanks to its polyphenols, and it outperforms many refined seed oils in cooking tests. The smoke point isn't the only factor to consider – what really matters is oxidative stability, and this is where olive oil wins. So, don't be afraid to roast or fry with EVOO.

What's wrong with seed oils?

This is one of the most hotly debated subjects on the internet when it comes to health, and I'm going to start by saying I'm not here to settle the debate.

There are two schools of thought: one is that seed oils are healthy and the other is that seed oils are a UPF and not healthy. There is evidence backed by credible doctors, nutritionists and health professionals to support BOTH sides of this argument.

For decades sunflower, rapeseed, and corn oils have been heralded as 'heart-healthy' as well as being neutral in flavour and cheap. Naturally, they took over our supermarket shelves. But there's no getting away from the fact that most of these oils are highly refined. This means the oil is extracted from the seeds at very high temperatures in a process, which often requires the use of chemical solvents, bleaching with adsorbent clays and deodorising to remove their naturally unpleasant smell. The result is a clear oil with a long shelf life but less nutritional value.

The worry is that this process not only strips flavour but also damages the delicate polyunsaturated fats that are naturally part of the oil, making them more prone to oxidation. Once oxidised, oils form harmful compounds called aldehydes which have been linked to systemic inflammation, atherosclerosis (furring of the arteries), and even DNA damage.

Another problem with seed oils is their omega-6 content. Omega-6 is an essential fatty acid, but it needs to be balanced with omega-3 to work well in the body. The ideal balance is from around 1:1 to 4:1. Because these cheap UPF seed oils crop up in or on so many foods, most people in the UK are consuming far too much and their omega-6 to omega-3 ratio is upwards of 20:1. That's a problem because excess omega-6 fuels inflammation and is linked to everything from heart disease to depression.

UPF seed oils are used in most packaged and UPF foods like crisps, takeaways, sauces, and salad dressings – so your exposure can add up fast. That's why I'm so keen to persuade people to check the labels on the food they buy and avoid their exposure to seed oils.

The seed oil debate is just going to rumble on because the only way to prove who is right would be to lock two people in a room and feed one of them seed oils while the other gets extra virgin olive oil. For quite a long time. Then measure their health parameters.

But one aspect on which the studies and scientists do agree unilaterally is that EVOO is the healthiest oil of all because it is such a rich source of beneficial plant compounds called polyphenols. So, in my opinion, there's no need to get involved in the whole messy seed oil debate. You have a clear choice: either save your money and accept a potential risk or invest a little extra money in your health and buy EVOO instead.

It's worth noting that seed oils in small amounts are not toxic, but the potential issue is cumulative exposure in modern diets as they are in almost everything. So, my advice would be to aim for EVOO but don't worry too much if seed oils have been snuck into some food that you eat while you are on the go and have no other choice.

	Extra virgin olive oil	Seed oils
How it's made	Cold-pressed, minimal processing.	Usually high-heat refined; many bleached/deodorised.
Fatty acid Profile	Mostly mono-unsaturated (~10% omega-6).	Higher omega-6 (Sunflower and soy: ~60–70%, Corn ~55–60%).

	Extra virgin olive oil	**Seed oils**
Antioxidants	High in polyphenols; strong antioxidant & anti-inflammatory effects.	Refining strips almost all polyphenols and vitamin E. Higher in antioxidents if cold pressed.
Cooking/ heat stability	Stable due to mono-unsaturated fats and antioxidants. Safe for sautéing/frying (180°C+).	High smoke points on paper, but oxidise more easily, producing aldehydes and peroxides.
Health outcomes	Strongest links to heart/brain benefits in Mediterranean diet.	Some evidence of benefit when replacing saturated fats, but less robust than EVOO. No polyphenol-linked protection.

Oils to invest in

Now, here's the good news. There are plenty of oils that don't just avoid harm, but they actively support your health. Let's break down the top four:

Extra virgin olive oil (EVOO)

This is the hero oil in any healthy kitchen. It's made by simply pressing olives – no chemicals, no high heat. That's why it's packed with antioxidants like polyphenols, which have been shown to lower inflammation, and protect against heart disease.

Use for: salads, roasting, stews, pasta, basically everything.

Avocado oil

Like olive oil, avocado oil is cold-pressed and rich in monounsaturated fats, which support heart health. Its smoke point is even higher than EVOO's, making it great for higher-heat cooking like stir fries.

Use for: frying, grilling, or when you need a neutral flavour.

Coconut oil

Coconut oil contains medium-chain triglycerides (MCTs), a unique fat that's quickly metabolised for energy. While traditional dietary guidelines recommend limiting saturated fat intake, a new meta-analysis of 26 studies found that the recommendation to avoid consuming coconut oil due to the risk of heart disease is not justified.[34]

Use for: baking, Asian dishes, occasional cooking.

Ghee

You've already read my take on butter, a great wholefood fat, especially when it's grass-fed. But if you want to cook at higher heat, ghee (clarified butter) is an underrated gem. It's got a high smoke point, no lactose, and is rich in fat-soluble vitamins.

Use for: sautéing, frying, roasting – when you want a heat-stable, nutrient-rich, aromatic fat.

Quick swap guide

Here's your quick checklist to get your oils right. If you've got some of these in the cupboard, it might be time for a swap:

SWAPS

Sunflower oil → Olive oil
If budget is tight, trade refined omega-6 seed oils for healthy monounsaturated fats or regular olive oil, which is roughly 30% cheaper than extra virgin.

Vegetable oil blends → Avocado oil
Higher monounsaturated fats and stable at high heat.

Olive oil → EVOO
It's definitely worth the investment if you can afford it. The dark green extra virgin is the real deal and comes with a host of polyphenols and antioxidants that are worth the investment.

Refined rapeseed oil → Cold-pressed rapeseed oil
If want to use rapeseed, choose the minimally processed version as it will be less oxidised and have more nutrients.

I appreciate extra virgin olive oil is expensive so if you need to save money on your olive oil, here's how to do it. Firstly, own-label olive oil is significantly cheaper (about 30% less) than branded and not necessarily worse quality.

I buy the single origin own-label organic, which I have found to be better than some brands. Another way to keep costs lower is invest in a spray bottle for your olive oil as this will ensure you don't use too much in cooking and can make your olive oil go further. One thing is clear: if you want to live longer, do as the Italians do and ensure you get lots of olive oil in your diet.

SWEET SPREADS

We've all stood in front of the spreads shelf, wondering what to slather on toast: a drizzle of honey? A spoonful of jam? Or a good dollop of peanut butter? Whichever is your favourite, there are good, bad and healthy options lined up right there in front of you.

> **THE GOOD**
> Raw honey from a single local source, 100% nut butters and homemade or reduced-sugar jams made with 70% whole fruit.
>
> **THE BAD**
> Chocolate or Biscoff spread, cheap jams with more sugar than fruit, honey 'blends' from multiple countries, and nut butters padded with palm oil and sugar.
>
> **THE HEALTHY**
> Pure honey, high-fruit-content jams (50%+ fruit), and nut butters with no palm oil or sugar.

Honey

Honey has been used as a sweetener for over 8,000 years, with ancient Egyptians offering it to their gods and even using it to dress wounds thanks to its natural antibacterial properties. A good-quality honey will contain trace minerals, enzymes, and antioxidants. That said, it's still high in natural sugar, so think of it as a healthier treat, not a free pass. Avoid honey blends that could have been fraudulently blended with sugar syrup. Honey fraud is surprisingly common, with cheap imports sometimes bulked out with sugar syrups to stretch supply. This doesn't make them unsafe, but it does mean you may be paying for something that's more glucose than golden honey. A jar of raw British honey will cost more but give you the genuine article, unprocessed and bursting with natural flavour.

Jam

Jam is a British classic. It was considered such an essential comfort during WWII that the government created a National Jam Scheme to ensure supplies were produced and rationed to the public. But here's the reality: many supermarket jars are 60% sugar – MORE sugar than fruit! A better choice, if you can afford it, is picking a jam with higher fruit content because this inevitably means it will contain less sugar. With more fruit in the jar, these jams actually taste better too. A word of caution: some brands try to trick you by using apple juice concentrate instead of refined sugar, allowing them to make the claim of 'no added sugar' or '100% fruit' – but the sugar content will still be high from juice rather than refined sugar.

Nut butter

Though Americans might claim to have invented peanut butter, it was a Canadian, Marcellus Edson, who first patented a peanut paste in 1884. Nut butters are the most nutritious of the bunch if you choose the right one. A jar of pure peanut, almond, or cashew butter gives you protein, fibre and healthy fats. It will also keep you feeling fuller for longer and can be a great breakfast or snack base. Always flip the jar and check the ingredients – it should just say nuts and salt. Avoid the brands that add palm oil or sugar to make them spread more evenly.

Chocolate spread

Now, I'm sure most of you know that Nutella isn't healthy, despite the manufacturer's best efforts to market it as a breakfast food. That jar of chocolate hazelnut spread is 56% sugar, and only 13% nuts, making it more a confectionery than a breakfast choice. If you can't resist that chocolate hit, have a look for nut butters blended with cocoa to deliver the same indulgent flavour but with far more protein, fibre, and healthy fats. Some contain only 9% sugar and over 63% nuts.

SWAPS

Cheap 'honey blend' → Raw or local honey
Less chance of fraud, cleaner, richer in antioxidants.

Standard jam → High-fruit jam or reduced-sugar conserve
Flavour from fruit, not spoonfuls of sugar.

Nut butters with palm oil → 100% nut butters
Healthier fats, no additives.

Chocolate hazelnut spreads → Pure nut butters with cocoa
Still indulgent, but higher in protein and lower in sugar.

If you stock your cupboard with 100% nut butters, raw honey and reduced-sugar, high-fruit jams, you can keep enjoying all the comfort of sourdough toast and spreads while sidestepping the worst offenders. These swaps don't just cut hidden sugars and additives, they also add a bit of real nutrition back into the mix. No need to banish these foods if you choose the versions that work with your health rather than against it.

THE SPICE RACK

A pinch of spice can transform the plainest dish into something delicious. From curry powder to smoked paprika, spices bring warmth, colour, and depth to meals. They're also one of the cheapest and healthiest ways to boost flavour.

And the best part? These health boosters cost pennies per teaspoon and add no sugar or unwanted nasties to your food.

If you're cooking a bit more from scratch (and I really hope I'm inspiring you to experiment with different foods and flavours), you might be intrigued by the vast array of options lined up on the supermarket spice rack. It can be very tempting to reach for the ready-made rubs and marinades with familiar labels such as 'fajita seasoning' or 'cajun mix' promising to make your food taste more 'Nandos'. But these blends are often made from different chemical flavourings and additives that mean you end up sprinkling UPF toxins over your lovingly prepared food.

It's also worth checking the price per 100g too. Spice mixes might look cheap, but they're often padded with salt, sugar, or maltodextrin and these low-cost fillers inflate the weight. This means you're paying more per gram of real spice than if you bought the pure jars individually.

Go for pure, single-ingredient jars and make your own blends instead. You'll unlock the genuine health benefits of spices, elevate your cooking, and avoid the sneaky additives hiding in the mixes. I urge you to look beyond the labelled jars and sachets, because the spice rack really is one supermarket aisle where you can genuinely 'season your way' to better health. A few basics in your cupboard will stretch further, taste better, and save you money over time.

The spice trade was once so valuable it literally shaped the world. In the 15th century, nutmeg was worth more than gold, and the search for pepper routes helped trigger the Age of Exploration. Fast forward to today and spices are among the most antioxidant-rich foods we can buy.

Cloves, cinnamon, oregano, turmeric and cumin all rank at the very top of antioxidant charts, which means they contain properties that have been shown to help reduce inflammation and protect cells from damage. Studies even suggest turmeric's active compound, curcumin, can support joint and brain health. Turmeric, cinnamon and cloves, for instance, score sky-high on the ORAC scale (a measure of antioxidant power), beating so-called superfoods such as blueberries hands down.

THE GOOD

Single spices (turmeric, cinnamon, cumin, paprika).
Pure, powerful and packed with antioxidants.

THE BAD

Cheap spice mixes or BBQ rubs where maltodextrin
or sugar is the first ingredient on the list.

THE HEALTHY

DIY blends: a mix of cumin, paprika, oregano and garlic powder to sprinkle on any dish. You'll cut hidden sugars, save money, and boost health benefits.

SWAPS

Fajita mix (sugar/maltodextrin first) → DIY fajita blend
Paprika, cumin, garlic, onion powder.

Curry powder (high in salt) → Turmeric with garam masala
Control the salt, keep the antioxidants.

BBQ rub (sugar-loaded) → Smoked paprika with chilli flakes
Smoky heat without the hidden teaspoons of sugar.

BISCUITS AND CRACKERS

The good old-fashioned biscuit has become an institution in the UK for dunking in a nice cup of tea, but its origins aren't British at all. The word biscuit comes from the Medieval Latin words *bis coctus* meaning twice cooked. In fact, early Roman biscuits were essentially bits of bread re-baked to make them crisp, which were then served as long-life, easy-to-transport rations.

The tradition eventually made it over to the British Isles and records in Scotland show 'biscuit bread' as early as the 12th century. However, in the 16th century biscuits were transformed into a luxurious treat when sugar and large amounts of butter were added to the dough. Mary, Queen of Scots, is credited with popularising what we now know as shortbread.

From chocolate chip cookies to the humble digestive, biscuits have become a staple part of our British culture. But with modern mass-production, our tastes have evolved, so that our favourite biscuits today are little more than a quick-hit ultra-processed sugar bomb. There could be as much as two teaspoons of sugar in some biscuits, which is bad enough, but can you ever be sure you'll stop at eating just one?

Luckily, I've been investigating healthier ways to dunk.

THE GOOD
Rich tea light (12% sugar, just 1.1g per biscuit),
the lowest-sugar dunker around.

THE BAD
Freshly baked cookies (40%+ sugar or 6+ teaspoons
each) and chocolate chip cookies (34%), which are
essentially sugar bombs disguised as biscuits.

THE HEALTHY
Plain classics like digestives (15% sugar) and
shortbread (17%), which keep sugar closer to
half a teaspoon per biscuit.

Here's a rundown of the options.

- Freshly baked cookies: 40% sugar, 27g per 66g cookie, which is over 6 teaspoons of sugar. Their high sugar content and their large size mean they are best avoided.
- Chocolate chip cookies: 34% sugar, 8.6g per 25g cookie, which is the equivalent of over 2 teaspoons of sugar – delicious, but there are better options.
- Chocolate digestives: 28% sugar, 4.8g per 16.7g biscuit, which is a teaspoon per biscuit (and I'm definitely not just eating one!).
- Shortbread: 17% sugar, 2.6g per shortbread – almost half a chocolate digestive.
- Digestive biscuits: 15% sugar, 2.2g per 15g biscuit. This is starting to look a lot healthier as we are only talking half a teaspoon of sugar per biscuit.

- Rich tea biscuits: 18% sugar, 1.5g per 8.3g biscuit. A healthier dunker due to the size. But the king of dunkers comes with Rich Tea's own 30% less sugar variety, which sits at 12% sugar and just 1.1g per biscuit, just a quarter of a teaspoon of sugar per biscuit.

So, when it comes to healthy dunking, the rich tea light biscuit is hard to beat. Its low sugar content and perfect dunkability make it a winner for health-conscious tea drinkers. Digestive biscuits are also a solid choice, especially if you prefer a bit more substance with your tea. For those moments when only chocolate will do, chocolate digestives are a good option although they do have a higher sugar content.

SWAPS

Freshly baked cookie (27g sugar) → Shortbread Finger (2.6g sugar)
Keep the indulgence but cut sugar by 90%.

Chocolate digestive (28% sugar) → Plain digestive (15% sugar)
Still satisfying, with half the sugar.

Chocolate chip cookie (8.6g sugar) → Rich tea light (1.1g sugar)
Save over 1.5kg sugar a year if you eat just four biscuits a week.

If you're looking to save money, own-brand biscuits from major supermarkets often offer comparable taste at

30%-50% discount on average, but rich tea and digestives are usually the best value per 100g.

So next time you need a tea break with a bit of a dunk, choose wisely and reduce your sugar intake significantly. If you eat just four biscuits a week, swapping from chocolate chip cookies to rich tea light could save you over 1.5kg of sugar per year from your diet. Small changes make a big impact.

The crack on crackers

Crackers feel like the sensible healthier alternative to biscuits if you are looking for pick-me-up snack or an evening nibble with cheese. But many crackers are ultra-processed, packed with flavour enhancers, sugars and with more salt than a bag of crisps. Old-school Ryvita and oatcakes are often the better options because they keep the ingredients simple and additives minimal. You can find sourdough crackers now in some stores, and these are also a great option.

Look at these ingredients for comparison:

Ryvita: *Wholegrain rye flour, rye flour, salt.*

Ritz Original Crackers: *Wheat flour, sunflower oil, sugar, glucose-fructose syrup, raising agents, salt, barley malt flour.*

A few crackers won't make or break your diet but it's good to watch out for these small areas of your food intake because that's where the junk can start creeping in. It's always worth swapping for the healthier option if you can.

SWAPS

Creams crackers → Wholegrain oatcakes
More fibre, less UPF.

Flavoured crackers → Rye crispbreads
Fewer ingredients, more fibre.

Selection boxes → Sourdough crackers
Fewer ingredients, easier to digest and healthier for you.

CRISPS

Who doesn't love a good crisp? That satisfying crunch is so addictive! Many people put themselves into a sweet or savoury category and, if you haven't got a particularly sweet tooth, I'll bet you're hooked on salty, crunchy snacks.

If you're the sort who simply can't stop at one, it might be reassuring to know it's not entirely your fault. Neuroscientists have found that the loud, crisp-breaking sound lights up the reward centres in our brain. They think this is because a crunch is associated with freshness and an intense eating experience. Studies show that the louder and crisper the sound when you bite, the fresher and tastier your brain perceives the food to be.

But at the same time, that clever combination of fat, salt and a rapid carbohydrate release triggers the release of dopamine, the feelgood hormone, which reinforces the pleasure and makes us reach for more. That crunch means that every mouthful stays novel and exciting, and this 'sensory-specific satiety' drives us to keep eating past the point of feeling full.

You don't need me to tell you that crisps are fundamentally unhealthy. There's no skirting the fact that most are UPF monstrosities packed with artificial flavourings, masses of salt, and deep fried in refined vegetable oils. The scary part is that, if you take the number of packs of crisps sold each year and divide it by the population, we are talking around 140 packs per person per year. This is a huge problem for our health.

But here's the healthy truth: you don't have to completely ditch the pleasure of a tasty, salty, crunchy snack IF you make healthier choices. Not all crisps are created equal and we're about to dive into the crisp aisle with a mission: finding the tastiest options that are kinder to your body.

THE GOOD

Alternatives like baked cheese, Snack A Jacks, baked pretzels, or even nuts and seeds. A big change from a standard crisp but one worth making.

THE BAD

Standard fried crisps with 30%+ fat content, fried in refined vegetable oils that oxidise under high heat.

THE HEALTHY

Small bags of lower-fat crispy snacks such as oven-baked crisps, popped chips, or popcorn. They give you the crunch without an excess oil load.

The great crisp conundrum: how to choose a healthier crunch

Here are three simple ways to make healthier choices when you shop the crisps aisle:

1. Understand the fat facts

Typical crisps are oil sponges that soak up the low-quality vegetable oils that have been heated to temperatures that oxidise the fat, increasing oxidative stress and inflammation within the body. It's easy to underestimate just how much fat you consume when you eat crisps. One standard bag contains around a tablespoon of oil. Eat a bag a day and that's over 2 litres of low-quality vegetable oil per year – and most of it oxidised from frying. Yuck! So, look out for crispy snacks that stay away from, or limit, the fat. Check the label and aim for anything that contains less than 15% total fat.

2. Fibre up your snack time

There's no escaping the fact that crispy snacks won't make a significant contribution to your nutritional intake, but it's worth checking the labels for fibre and protein as some are most definitely better than others. For instance, plain popcorn still comes in with a fat content of 17.4%, but you do get double the fibre of standard crisps at 10.9g per 100g. This is where lentil crisps are also a great option, with only 18% fat and 4x more fibre and 6x more protein than standard crisps.

This will not only help you feel fuller for longer, but also help to keep your digestive system happy, reducing the chance of overeating.

3. Apply portion control

Let's be real – we've all managed to demolish a family-sized 'sharing bag' on our own in one sitting. If you know you struggle to stop when you've started, it's a good idea to just stop buying the big bags. Many brands offer multi-pack bags that are portion-controlled, usually around 25g per bag. This helps manage intake and prevents overindulging.

SWAPS

Big sharing bags → Multipack mini bags (25g)
Built-in portion control prevents overindulgence.

Standard Walkers (30% fat) → Walkers oven baked or popped chips (13% fat)
Same crunch, half the oil.

Crisps → Snack A Jacks (8.3% fat)
Rice cake crunch, a third of the fat at 8.3% fat per 100g.

Crisps → Baked pretzels (4.6% fat)
The lowest-fat crisp alternative option at only 4.6% fat per 100g.

Crisps → Nuts/seeds/dried cheese
Packed with protein and good fats for satiety.

Want to be even healthier? Switch to nuts, seeds or even dried cheese snacks. They might be higher in calories, but you get protein, fibre, nutrients and good healthy fats, all of which makes them more satiating and limits the chance of overeating.

With these tips, you can pick smarter, snack better, and still satisfy those crunchy cravings. If you're the sort to grab a bag of crisps each day as part of your 'meal deal' lunch, and you make some of my swaps instead, you could be cutting a crazy 2 litres of oil from your diet over the course of the year.

Disclaimer: I'm definitely not giving you permission to eat crisps every day! This is just an illustration of how small changes add up quickly overtime. Go ahead and enjoy a bag of crisps as an occasional treat instead. Happy snacking!

CHOCOLATE AND SWEETS

Time for the chocolate aisle – a marketer's dream of childhood nostalgia, bright colours, silver-and-gold wrapped bars all formulated and packaged with nothing but pure pleasure in mind. Sooooo unhealthy you might think! But the bittersweet irony here is that what is considered as one of the unhealthiest aisles in the store is actually one of the healthiest.

For most of history, chocolate wasn't a sweet treat at all. The ancient Mayans and Aztecs drank cacao as a bitter, spiced drink, often mixed with chilli and water, believing it to be a gift from the gods (that would be a superfood in our language today).

Superfoods now come with a premium price tag more expensive than champagne. They are like designer outfits that look dazzling on the runway but somehow lose their sparkle on a Friday night at Wetherspoons. They have exotic names and promise health benefits that are rarely backed up by science, and anyway the quantities are usually too small to make any impact on your health.

But what if there was a way to get your hands on more antioxidants than any superfood can provide? In its purest form, cacao is still one of the most antioxidant-rich foods on earth. It has over 40 times more health-giving antioxidants than blueberries. It wasn't until sugar was added to cacao in 16th-century Europe that chocolate was born, and then, in the last century more sugar, milk powders and vegetable oils have been routinely added to tip our beloved chocolate into being a UPF indulgence.

The great chocolate classics of Galaxy, Dairy Milk, Mars Bars and KitKats are comfortingly familiar. They are everywhere. You can't escape them in the supermarket – in multi-buy offers, by the till, in lunchbox multipacks. They're cheap, they're heavily marketed as family-friendly, and they hit that all-important 'bliss factor' of sugar with fat that lights up our pleasure centres perfectly and makes them almost impossible to resist.

The problem? These bars are more than 50% sugar, and it is that sugar content that leads to sugar crashes, overindulgence and poor teeth, especially in children. White chocolate is even higher in sugar too. The worst I've seen is 63% sugar in a bar of chocolate. And that's why we need to make a swap.

THE GOOD

Dark chocolate 85 – 90% cocoa solids. Rich in antioxidants, dramatically lower in sugar – as little as 7g per 100g bar. Ideally organic.

THE BAD

Standard milk chocolate: often contains only 25% cocoa solids, bulked out with sugar at crazy levels. Don't get me started on white chocolate! These are more confectionery than cacao.

THE HEALTHY
Dark chocolate with anything over 70% cocoa solids
which delivers antioxidants, magnesium, iron, and
flavanols that support heart and brain health.

Here's the difference broken down:

Chocolate (cocoa solid content)	Approx sugar (per 100g)
Milk (25%)	54g
Dark (47%)	49g
Dark (70%)	29g
Dark (85%)	15g
Dark (90%)	7g

Chocolate: your surprise superfood

Typically, superfood green powders that you are supposed to stir into smoothies will set you back anywhere from £50-£2,000 per kg depending on the brand. The different blends of plants such as spirulina and wheatgrass often promise eternal youth, but in reality, many provide a blend of greens that have limited scientific evidence to support any of their specific benefit claims. They are little more than a glorified multivitamin.

This is where dark chocolate steps in as a real superfood. Gram for gram, cocoa can pack more antioxidant punch than wheatgrass and even blueberries. It delivers minerals like magnesium, iron, potassium, and copper, which are essential for muscles, nerves, and energy. The polyphenols, especially flavanols and epicatechins, support blood flow, reduce oxidative stress, and help protect your cells. On top of that, cocoa naturally contains dietary fibre, so each square supports gut health by feeding friendly bacteria.

Choose high-cocoa, low-sugar dark chocolate and you are not just indulging, you are getting real nutritional benefits, while supermarket chocolate tends to come in at only £25-35 per kg, which is almost half the price of your cheapest green powder. If you are anything like me, a couple of squares after dinner each night goes down a treat, which means you'll be knocking back 200g of superfood chocolate a week.

Train your taste buds

The good news is that there is a way to indulge in chocolate daily to create a superfood routine without the sugary side effects. And even if you think you're a milk chocaholic and you can't bear the bitter taste of dark chocolate, I'm going to show you how to learn to love this delicious powerhouse of health.

It is possible to re-train your taste buds in just 10 days to get the superfood benefits of 85% and above. The trick is to start at the lower percentages and then gradually work your way up to the darker percentages. Get to a level you are comfortable with and then make sure you have a piece of chocolate every night for 10 days straight. That's my prescription to you! Believe me, after 10 days your taste buds will adapt, and you will be able to take the next step up to a darker chocolate. Repeat the same process at the next level. Take it step by step and you'll be able to go all the way to 90% dark. That's what my three-year-old son enjoys regularly, so if he can do it, I believe you can too.

The switch from milk chocolate to 70% dark will save you 2.6kg of sugar a year, while working your way up to 90% will save you over 4.8kg of sugar per year (assuming 200g consumption per week). Training your taste buds takes a bit of work, but in return you get huge sugar savings that are worth it not just for the reduction in sugar but also the increase in antioxidants.

You can see from the table below that the more you train your taste buds, the less sugar you consume.

SWAPS

Green powders → Cacao powder
For smoothies and baking, cacao offers more antioxidants at half the price of spirulina or wheatgrass.

Milk chocolate (25% cocoa, 54g sugar) → 70% dark (29g sugar)
Halve your sugar intake and double your antioxidants.

70% dark → 85% dark
An easy next step to cut sugar almost in half again (from 29g to 15g per 100g).

85% dark → 90% dark
Reduce sugar to just 7g per 100g while maximising antioxidants.

Skip the sharing bags

Movie night, when we're tucked up together with the kids nice and cozy on the sofa, is one of my favourites. Amid all the chaos of parenting, this is a lovely moment of calm for the family. We all love a good movie and the pleasure is usually enhanced by some sweet treats to nibble on.

I reckon that's what the family-friendly chocolate sharing bags, which were launched in the late 1990s, were created for – it's a brilliant bit of marketing to create a new chocolate-based ritual to boost sales. But my worry is the studies which show that over a third of 16-24 year olds don't share these bags at all.[35] Then when you notice the way that some manufacturers *increase* the sugar content in sharing bags compared to their usual packs and bars to make them cheaper, it means a massive sugar bomb on movie night. It makes me realise there might be a problem here we need to address.

THE GOOD

Skip the sharing bag altogether and hand out high-cocoa dark chocolate bars of 85%+. You can break them up into squares and freeze or refrigerate them.

THE BAD

The big-brand milk chocolate bags such as M&Ms and Galaxy Counters are cheap, packed with unnecessary sugar and very easy to overconsume.

> **THE HEALTHY**
> Pick out lower-sugar options or something with a
> higher cocoa content, such as Dark Maltesers. They
> still feel indulgent but slash sugar nearly in half
> compared to the worst offenders.

Making the right chocolate choices can drastically cut your sugar intake without spoiling the fun. Let's dive into the world of chocolate sharing bags and discover how you can enjoy a treat while being kinder to your health.

- M&Ms – 66% sugar
- Galaxy Counters – 58% sugar
- Cadbury Buttons – 56% sugar
- Reese's Mini Cups – 54% sugar
- Regular Maltesers – 53% sugar
- Maltesers Dark Chocolate – 32% sugar

The truth is, cocoa is expensive and sugar is cheap. So 'value' bigger packs will be loading you with sugar.

The NHS daily recommendation for sugar intake is 30g a day for adults, 24g a day for seven to 10-year-olds, and 19g a day for four to six-year-olds. But a 125g bag of M&Ms delivers an astounding 82.5 grams of sugar per bag. That's over 20 teaspoons of sugar or 2.75x of your daily recommended intake for adults in just one bag – and we all know that one bag never makes it through movie night unfinished.

Now let's look at the health champion in the list – Maltesers Dark Chocolate. At just 32% sugar in an 88g bag, we are talking about a cool 28 grams of sugar per bag. That's still 7 teaspoons of sugar and 93% of your daily sugar allowance but it's a whopping 65% less sugar than M&Ms – so that's a big win for your health.

SWAPS

Large family sharing bag → Mini multipack bags
Portion control by design helps avoid demolishing a big bag in one go.

Sharing bags → Regular chocolate bars
Ditch the endless grazing for a few squares. The portion control will help and simple chocolate bars are often lower in sugar.

Regular Maltesers (53% sugar) → Dark Maltesers (32% sugar)
Same brand, better choice.

M&Ms (66% sugar) → Dark Maltesers (32% sugar)
A 65% sugar saving per bag.

Now if you have one movie night a week (around 60 per year) snuggled up on the sofa and enjoying those chocolatey treats, then switching from M&Ms to Dark Maltesers could give you a massive 3.2 kilo grams of sugar savings per year. The cost is the same, but the Maltesers bag is 30% smaller and your health will certainly thank you. When it comes to sweet treats, portion control is important.

If Maltesers aren't quite your thing, just switch to dark chocolate bars with a high cocoa content (85% or higher), as these have much less sugar and more beneficial antioxidants.

Sweets for your sweeties

We all love a sweet treat once in a while, and there's nothing you're going to be able to do to stop kids wanting sweets. But you might be surprised to learn that some are definitely healthier than others, and I've got some clever swaps up my sleeve that could slash your sugar intake by 50%.

It is important to point out that a typical 100g of sweets might contain 40-70g of sugar, which could double your child's daily sugar limit in one swift hit.

THE GOOD

Small bags or portion controlled lower-sugar options with natural ingredients such as Haribo Fruitilicious multipacks which deliver less sugar and fewer additives.

THE BAD

Sugar bombs like Skittles (74% sugar), Haribo Supermix (55%), and Tangfastics (50%).

THE HEALTHY

Haribo Zingfest (32% sugar) or Rowntrees Berry Hearts (35% sugar). These still feel like a treat but cut sugar almost in half compared to Skittles.

Let's start with the worst offenders: Skittles. These colourful candies claim that you can taste the rainbow, but they pack a whopping 74% sugar which leaves little room to taste anything but the sugar. To put that into perspective, that's almost three-quarters of each Skittle being pure sugar and you chomp through 25 teaspoons of sugar in one 136g bag. This sugar hit can wreak havoc on your health and the multitude of artificial colours just makes things worse.

No one would try to convince you that Haribo is healthy, but whether you're partial to the sour tang of Tangfastics or the variety of Starmix, this does provide an opportunity to cut your sugar intake in dramatically:

- **Supermix** takes the sugar crown with 55% sugar.
- **Tangfastics** with their sugary coating are sadly one of the worst with 50% sugar content.
- **Starmix** without the sugar coating helps bring the content down to 47%.
- **Fruitilicious** is a fruity option with 34% sugar content.
- **Zingfest** may not be the name you immediately think of when you think of Haribo, but these guys are my new favourite with only 32% sugar.

The difference becomes clear when you break that down into teaspoons of sugar. A 175g Supermix sharebag delivers 24 teaspoons of sugar but a 150g Zingfest sharebag has only 12 teaspoons. That's a massive 50% reduction in your sugar content just by swapping Haribos. Yes, it's a smaller bag size but portion control is important when you can be sure no one is going to be putting an already opened bag back in the cupboard.

SWAPS

Sharing bags → Mini packs
Built-in portion control to avoid demolishing
20+ teaspoons of sugar in one sitting.

**Skittles (74% sugar) → Rowntree's Berry Hearts
(35% sugar)**
Cut sugar in half in one simple swap.

**Haribo Supermix (55% sugar) → Haribo Zingfest
(32% sugar)**
Same Haribo, different health effect.

If I ate sweets, I'd be quite excited by Rowntree's Berry Hearts. These little heart-shaped gummies not only do my taste buds a favour by getting rid of all the yellows and oranges in favour of a bag full of reds and purples, but at 35% their sugar content is relatively low. Even better is the attempt to reduce the artificial additives and colourings – they use black carrot, carrot and hibiscus to colour the sweets.

If you give your kids a bag of Skittles every week you're notching up over 5.2kg of extra sugar a year. Swapping to Berry Hearts saves over 3kg of sugar (2.1kg a year). Even when indulging in sweets, opting for those with lower sugar content can make a big difference. Stay sweet but keep it healthy!

COFFEE AND TEA

The smell of fresh coffee first thing in the morning or the warming comfort of a hot cup of tea are all part of important daily rituals for many of us. The good news is that coffee and tea are a great source of antioxidants, which means they can be brilliant for your health, helping to improve focus, and even reducing the risk of certain diseases. In fact, studies have even found that coffee is the number one source of antioxidants in many people's diets. But the benefits you glean will depend entirely on how you drink your chosen brew – add too much sugar, syrups, or cream, and your 'healthy pick-me-up' can quickly become a dessert in disguise.

THE GOOD
Fairtrade, organic freshly ground beans brewed at home, and plastic-free or loose-leaf teas. Full flavour, antioxidants, no hidden sugars or plastics.

THE BAD
Flavoured instant sachets with sugar as the first ingredient, plastic pod systems that leach microplastics, and nylon tea bags shedding billions of plastic particles per brew.

THE HEALTHY
Any plain coffee or tea is antioxidant-rich and healthy.

Caffeine, the natural stimulant in coffee and tea, can be beneficial in moderation, boosting concentration and even mood. Researchers have noted that a moderate coffee intake of one or two cups a day is associated with health benefits and may help ward off health issues. The key lies in that word 'moderation'. In this range, you reap the benefits without overdoing the caffeine. Tea typically contains less caffeine than coffee, so you can go ahead and enjoy a few cups of tea throughout the day without worrying about its impact on your nerves or sleep. And unlike coffee, tea naturally contains l-theanine, an amino acid that promotes relaxation and steadies the caffeine effect, which is why a cuppa tends to feel more calming despite the caffeine it contains.

If you're sensitive to caffeine, it's good to know just how little it takes to affect your sleep. Caffeine has a half-life of five or six hours, which means your 3pm coffee will still be trickling caffeine into your system at bedtime, potentially disrupting deep sleep even if you find you drift off easily. Poor sleep in turn worsens hunger hormones, making you more likely to crave sugar and caffeine the next day.

The solution is simple. Enjoy coffee in the morning or just after lunch but stick to tea through the afternoon. That way you get the best of both worlds: energy by day, rest by night.

The heathiest way to take your coffee is freshly brewed through a basic drip filter, a cafetière or a pour-over coffee maker. This way you'll be getting pure coffee and water, without any of the artificial additives, sugars, or plastics that can come with pods or machines that run hot water through plastic pipes.

For the ultimate cup, look out for Fairtrade-certified and organic coffee. A fairtrade stamp ensures the farmers who grew your beans were paid fairly and it often means there has been support offered to aid community development. Organic coffee is also worth paying for if you can. Coffee is one of the most chemically treated crops in the world. Traces of those agrochemicals can remain on the beans. At low levels, these will be unlikely to affect your health in the short term but, as I've repeatedly pointed out throughout this book – every little counts. And if you buy fairtrade coffee you will be supporting farming practices that are better for the environment and farm workers' health. In my opinion, that's worth it, if you can afford it.

Beware the fancy coffees

Nestling among the packs and jars of coffee beans and powders on the supermarket shelves, you'll also find an array of instant coffee mixes, pods, and canned coffee drinks promising café-style flavour in a flash. Unfortunately, many of these products are super-powered by unwanted additives. The worst offenders are the instant latte/cappuccino sachets. If you check the ingredients, you might be shocked to see sugar listed first – ahead of coffee, which makes up around 12% of the contents. Tip one into a cup and pour over boiling water and you will be drinking a hot cup of sugar with a hint of coffee.

Toxic pods

Another modern convenience that carries a hidden downside is coffee pods. Many single-serve coffee machines brew coffee in plastic capsules. These pods are incredibly handy: pop them into the machine, press a button, and you have a consistently delicious cup of coffee. But have you stopped for a minute to consider what hot water pumping through a plastic pod might do? Research suggests that brewing coffee in plastic single-use pods can cause microplastic particles to leach into your drink as the combination of boiling water, high pressure, and acidic coffee draws out tiny plastic fragments from the capsule. Aluminium capsules are better for the environment and better for you.

Time for tea

Tea has a cherished place in British culture; there's nothing like a hot cuppa to soothe the soul. The wonderful thing about tea is that, whether you favour the classic English breakfast or a herbal infusion, you'll be getting a beverage that's hydrating and often rich in antioxidants. Regular tea drinking has been linked to a host of potential benefits, from lower risk of heart disease to improved gut health.

You won't find the same nutritional red flags with tea that you do with fancy coffees because tea is typically consumed plain or with just a dash of milk (and maybe a spoonful of sugar). The one surprising caution with tea is not about what's in the leaves but what's in the tea bags. You might assume a tea bag is just paper, but many modern tea bags (especially the fancy pyramid-shaped ones) actually contain plastic. Some tea bags are made from nylon or food-grade PET (a type of plastic) and others use polypropylene glue to seal the edges. When you pour boiling water over these bags, microplastics can shed into your brew. A startling study in 2019 found that a single plastic tea bag (steeped at typical brewing temperature) released about 11.6 billion microplastic particles into one cup of tea.[36]

The good news is that most UK tea brands have been responding to this issue and there's been a push for plastic-free, biodegradable tea bags. Several big brands now use compostable plant-fibre bags or have switched to designs that don't require plastic sealants. Pukka, Clipper, Teapigs, PG Tips and Yorkshire Tea have moved to fully biodegradable bags, and lots of others are following. To be on the safe side, you can look for brands that explicitly declare on the box that their bags are plastic-free. Alternatively, consider making your brew the old-fashioned way with loose leaf tea and a strainer or infuser. The bottom line: tea itself is a healthy drink, just keep an eye on the packaging.

SWAPS

Flavoured coffee sachets (e.g. vanilla latte mix) → Plain coffee

Supermarket sachets often have sugar as the first
ingredient; plain coffee lets you add your own milk
or flavouring without hidden sugars.

Instant coffee → Ground coffee

Instant contains higher levels of acrylamide
(a compound formed in processing), while brewed
ground coffee has less.

Plastic pods → Aluminium pods

Aluminium pods don't leach microplastics when
hot water runs through, and most are now recyclable.

Ground coffee → Whole beans

Whole beans keep fresher for longer since less
surface area is exposed to oxygen. Grind at home
for a richer, more aromatic cup.

Budget coffee → Fairtrade/organic coffee

Supermarket fairtrade or organic lines cost a little
more but avoid pesticide residues and support
better farming standards.

Plastic-based pyramid tea bags → Plastic-free tea bags

Choose brands that now label their bags
'plastic-free' (e.g. PG Tips, Yorkshire Tea) to
avoid microplastics in your brew.

By making these simple swaps and being aware of what's
in your cup, you can continue to enjoy your coffee or
tea habit while maximising the health benefits and minimising any downsides. With a bit of modern knowledge,

you can sip smarter: revel in the rich antioxidants and comforting warmth, without the excess sugar, chemicals, or plastics. So, go ahead, put the kettle on and keep reading the rest of the book.

SOFT DRINKS

Ah, the soft drink aisle! This is where you'll find a technicolour wonderland of bubbles and promises and most likely some of the cause of the nation's diabetes issues! Studies consistently show a clear correlation[37] between the number of soft drinks consumed and the risk of getting type 2 diabetes. Those rows and rows of different flavours, tastes and colours are hiding kilos and kilos of sugar.

It is slightly ironic that soft drinks were originally created with a healthy intention. It was a pharmacist called John Pemberton who first created Coca-Cola in 1886 – and he wasn't the first. A Brooklyn-born pharmacist called Charles Alderton invented Dr Pepper in 1885, a drink that was initially designed and marketed as a digestive aid.

The multi-billion-pound drinks industry would like you to believe that the drinks themselves aren't really that bad. They say it's our fault for drinking too many of them.

Or is there something more sinister going on?

> ## THE BAD
> Standard fizzy drinks: Coca-Cola (35g sugar per can), Fanta, Sprite. Diet drinks which switch sugar for aspartame and acesulfame K aren't much better for your health.
>
> ## THE HEALTHY
> Look out for newer fizzy drink options such as gut health sodas and kombucha (fermented tea), which are lowering the sugar content of the soft drink industry.

Grown-up fizzy pop

A typical 330ml can of Coca-Cola packs 35g of sugar – that's nearly nine teaspoons in a single serving. The NHS recommends adults cap 'free sugars' at 30g a day, so that's your daily allowance (and then some) gone in three big gulps. This will spike you blood sugar significantly and will probably lead you to a sugar crash, which will see you reaching for the snacks in no time. The low-calorie bros will be shouting, 'Never fear, diet is here,' but diet drinks are no better. It's just a simple marketing trick, whereby they swap out the sugar for artificial sweeteners, aspartame and acesulfame K. There are thousands of scientific studies on the topic of whether artificial sweeteners are bad for your health. In my search, I found that 50% *conclusively* identified a negative association, while a further 23% *possibly* found a link, which would suggest over 73% of studies looking into artificial sweeteners found they pose an increasing risk of metabolic disease. We have to acknowledge that regulators still class them as safe, but these studies do raise red flags. It's up to you – it's your body and your choice whether you want to take the risk. Personally, I don't![38]

So, what's going on? It looks like artificial sweeteners might actually enhance sugar cravings rather than suppress them, so picking a 'diet' drink could lead to more snacking and over-consumption. These drinks have also been shown to alter the gut microbiome (the vast populations of bacteria which happily live in our gut) with potentially negative health effects.

OJ sugar bomb

There's a wolf hiding in sheep's clothes even in the seemingly innocent glass of orange juice. I'm a stickler for the sugars and a 300ml glass contains around 24g of sugar – that's six teaspoons, with none of the fibre of a whole orange to slow down the sugar rush. These liquid sugar bombs might taste good, but your blood glucose (and waistline) will be anything but good if you are necking the OJ regularly.

The whizz on energy drinks

I thought about leaving this section out of my book because by now you'll know a bit about me, and you have probably worked out that I think energy drinks like Red Bull and Monster are pretty bad. But given their ubiquitous availability and the fact that I still see people drinking them all the time, I thought it'd be worth a quick explanation as to why they are EVEN worse than cola. It's the combination of excessive sugar, artificial caffeine and taurine that delivers the desired energy rush. A single

250ml can of Red Bull contains around 27g of sugar (almost seven teaspoons) plus 80mg of caffeine, which is more than what you get in a single espresso.

Buy a super-sized 500ml can of Monster Energy and you get to double those figures. It's completely crazy that teenagers are buying these drinks. The sugar spikes your blood glucose, the caffeine overstimulates your nervous system, and when both wear off, you'll be left with a sharp crash. Regular consumption has been linked to poor sleep, anxiety, and weight gain.

So, what's the alternative? Do we need to banish all joy and drink water forever? Not quite. This is where some clever newer brands step in. Meet TRIP, a CBD-infused sparkling drink that's surprisingly low in sugar (around 5g per can). Dash Water is my absolute go-to right now. It's simply sparkling water infused with natural fruit flavour and here's the kicker: zero sugar, zero sweeteners, zero calories. It's hydration as it should be, water that will still give you that cold fizzy-can moment.

SWAPS

Coca-Cola (35g sugar) → TRIP (5g sugar)
Cut 30g sugar per can, and 1.5kg a year if you drink
one a week.

**Orange juice (24g sugar per glass) → Whole orange
(9g sugar + fibre)**
Swap liquid sugar for slower-release natural sugar
with fibre.

**Diet Coke (0g sugar + sweeteners) → Dash sparkling
water (0g sugar, no sweeteners)**
Avoid artificial additives entirely.

Want a homemade budget-friendly swap? Try infusing plain water with cucumber, mint or lemon. Add ice or make it fizzy with sparkling water. That's pennies saved per glass and you'll sidestep the sugar crash entirely.

The key takeaway here is simple:

- Watch for hidden sugars even in "natural" drinks like juice.
- Skip artificial sweeteners when you can – they're not the health halo they promise.
- Celebrate brands that keep it simple, such as Dash and TRIP, or DIY your hydration at home.

Because in the Wild West of adult drinks, being savvy means you can still sip something special, without the sugar hangover.

ALCOHOL

This chapter is dedicated to my dad, Mouni van Kampen, who loves a glass of wine. Or two. For years, I tried to get him to understand that the occasional tipple might be ok, but it's just not healthy to be necking two glasses of red wine every night. He was so stubborn. No matter how hard I preached the science and quoted the studies about accumulated health risks, he refused to listen.

The sobering truth is no amount of alcohol is healthy – that might be just as hard for you to swallow as it was for my dad. Alcohol is treated by the body as a toxin, which means the liver has to deal with it before almost anything else. This process stresses the body, disrupting blood sugar balance, raising blood pressure, and interfering with normal sleep. Over time, these effects add up. Large global studies, including one published in *The Lancet* (2018)[39] with over half a million participants, have shown that even small amounts of alcohol increase long-term risks of cancer, heart disease and liver problems and shorten life expectancy.

Eventually I realised that this wasn't down to a lack of knowledge or understanding on Dad's part, it was the psychological link between red wine and the taste of reward and pleasure at the end of a long working day. Dad worked very hard as a carpenter and he felt he deserved his glass of red wine (or two). He wasn't going to give up that sense of reward.

I needed to find a swap that would allow him to keep his moment of pleasure, but in a healthier way.

Believe me, he had every excuse, his favourite one being that we've drunk alcohol for thousands of years. Which is true. The earliest evidence of winemaking comes from clay jars in Georgia, dating back to 6000 BC. Ancient Egyptians brewed beer daily, and the Greeks saw wine as a gift from the gods. But it was also drunk as a safer alternative to water. The fermentation process killed off the potentially harmful bacteria that lurked in the water in those days, making it safer to choose alcohol over anything else.

Thankfully, those concerns no longer apply.

If you like a drink, or two, here's how to make smarter choices:

THE GOOD

Dry wines (pinot noir, sauvignon blanc, brut champagne) with minimal residual sugar, or simple spirits such as tequila, gin, or whisky served neat or with soda.

THE BAD

Sweet wines (port, moscato), sugary cocktails (margaritas, piña coladas), and standard G&Ts with full-sugar tonic.

THE HEALTHY

Anything that lowers the sugar content – choose pinot noir over malbec, vodka soda over cocktails, gin with light tonic, or hard seltzers with 1–2g sugar. You will still get an alcohol buzz, but with far less metabolic chaos.

But red wine is healthy, right?

For years, red wine enjoyed a bit of a health halo, thanks to the polyphenols such as resveratrol, which come from the skins of dark-coloured grapes. These compounds act as antioxidants, and early studies in the 1990s suggested they could help to protect the heart by improving blood flow and reducing inflammation.

But while polyphenols are real and healthy, the quantities you might get in a glass – or even a bottle – of wine are tiny. You'd need to drink dozens of glasses a day to reach the optimal levels required to have any kind of health effect, and any small benefit from those antioxidants will be far outweighed by the risks associated with drinking alcohol. The truth is, you can get way more polyphenols from eating grapes, blueberries, or even peanuts, without the downsides of alcohol.

The search for a healthier red wine

Wines can range from bone-dry, containing virtually no sugar, to dessert-sweet and loaded with the stuff. Ok, I'm being quite picky here, as some wine only has 2g of sugar per glass. That might not seem like a lot, but that sugar load can add up.

Let's take my dad as an example. He's 72. The average life expectancy in the UK for a man is 82. So, assuming he's got another ten years of drinking a couple of glasses of wine a night, the numbers will really stack up. At roughly 2g per glass of malbec, that's 4g of sugar per night, multiplied by 365 days a year over ten years, equals 14.6kg of sugar. Pinot noir is equally delicious, but has just 0.7-1g of sugar per glass on average. It does depend on the length of fermentation the specific winery uses. By making this easy switch, my dad's future possible wine sugar load could drop by half to 7.3kg. It's a worthwhile saving for him, but even better if you've got 40 good years of drinking left in you.

The fascinating truth is that some wines are sweeter than others. What drives this huge difference? It comes down to the natural grape sugars left over after fermentation. If yeast ferments all the sugar, you get a dry wine with minimal sweetness. But if the winemaker stops fermentation early, some sugar remains and the wine tastes sweeter.

So, a sweet wine such as port can pack almost three teaspoons (12g) of sugar per glass, and two glasses could deliver almost an entire day's recommended sugar limit.

My dad is very happy with pinot noir, and if I have the odd glass of wine when we are eating out, I'll pick pinot noir too, but check out the average sugar comparisons below:

Red wines (150ml)	Approx sugar (g)
Port (fortified sweet)	10–12g
Lambrusco (semi-sweet)	6g
Zinfandel (red, semi-sweet)	2–4g
Merlot	1–2g
Cabernet sauvignon	1–2g
Syrah/shiraz	1–2g
Malbec	1.5–2g
Pinot noir	0.7–1g

SWAPS

Malbec (2g) → Pinot noir (0.7-1g)
Halve sugar per glass over a decade of drinking.

Port (12g) → Dry red (1–2g)
Swap dessert wine for standard wine and
save 11g sugar per glass.

Riesling (6g) → Sauvignon blanc (1.5g)
Swap the sweeter varieties for dry, crisp and refreshing
whites that will cut your sugar intake per glass.

Sweet Zinfandel rosé (5g) → Dry Provençal rosé (2g)
It may be beautiful on a summers day but it's a sweet
treat that can be swapped for a Provençal to cut your
sugar per glass in half.

Prosecco dry (3-5g) → Prosecco brut (0-2g)
Same celebration, just with about half the sugar.

White wines and rosés

White / rosé (150ml)	Approx sugar (g)
Moscato (sweet white)	8g
Riesling (semi-sweet)	6g
White zinfandel (sweet rosé)	5g
Rosé (dry Provençal style)	2g
Sauvignon blanc (dry white)	1.5g
Chardonnay (dry white)	1.5g
Dry champagne/prosecco	3-5g
Brut champagne/prosecco	0-2g

The sugar content of white wines will vary more extensively than red. A crisp dry white (say a sauvignon blanc) might contain only 1.5g per glass, while an off-dry white such as riesling can be several grams higher. Rosé wines often fall in between but can surprise you: a sweet white zinfandel rosé could have around 5g per glass, whereas a dry rosé will be much lower.

But because wineries aren't required to put sugar content on labels, these differences aren't obvious from the bottle.

Be sure of sulphites

Sulphites are the preservatives used in wine-making to prevent oxidation and bacterial spoilage, which gives wine a longer shelf life. While most people tolerate sulphites just fine, you might notice headaches, nasal congestion, or skin flushing when you drink wine containing sulphites. Choosing sulphite-free or low-sulphite wines can reduce these potential reactions and it also means fewer additives in your glass. If you're aiming for a cleaner, more natural sip, try seeking out organic pinot noir with no added sulphites as it can be a gentler option on your body.

At the end of the day, alcohol is something to enjoy in moderation, and knowing the sugar content of your favourite tipple helps you drink more wisely because sugar and alcohol make the perfect hangover storm. When you combine alcohol with sugar, whether it's from sweet mixers or high-sugar wines, you're basically doubling down on dehydration and metabolic chaos. Sugar spikes your blood glucose, then crashes it, while alcohol is a diuretic that makes you lose even more fluids. Together, they stress your liver, pull water from your system, and amplify inflammation. This means a pounding head, dry mouth, and that dreaded hit-by-a-truck feeling the next day. Opting for lower-sugar drinks doesn't just help your sugar intake; it can make your morning-after far less brutal.

If wine isn't your thing, you can still make smarter choices when you're choosing what to drink. The good news is there are plenty of options for sensible sipping, which allow you to cut out excess sugar while still enjoying a boozy treat.

Lighter lagers

Beer is often left out of the sugar debate because it doesn't taste sweet, but it's loaded with carbohydrates that act like sugar in the body. A pint of lager has 180–200kcal and 15g carbs which is roughly the same carb impact as two or three slices of white bread. Over a week, a couple of pints a night habit could quietly add the equivalent of an extra loaf of bread to your diet.

SWAPS

Beer → Light beer

Lighter beers aren't just for taste; the lower alcohol content equals fewer carbs and calories for your body to deal with. You may think going from a 5% beer to a 4% is an insignificant difference but it's a 25% reduction in calories.

Beer → Alcohol-free beer

Same moment of enjoyment, but fewer calories and most importantly no alcohol.

Spirits

Vodka

Vodka or any pure spirit such as gin, rum or whisky, contains *virtually no sugar* on its own, but the devil lies in the sugary mixers like coke, lemonade and orange juice. But by mixing it with fizzy water and a squeeze of fresh lime or lemon, you add flavour without any added sugars. It's hydrating, simple, and arguably the cleanest cocktail you can order at a bar.

> **SWAPS**
>
> **Vodka Coke (25g+ of sugar) → Vodka soda with fresh lime (0g)**
> Same refreshing flavour without the sugar and you should feel better for it the next morning.

Hard seltzers

These are basically boozy sparkling waters, often naturally flavoured with fruit essence. In recent years, hard seltzers (or alcoholic sparkling waters) have become a go-to for those looking to 'drink light'. Many popular ones contain just 1–2g of total sugar per can – which is less sugar than even a dry wine or light beer in most cases, so makes for a better choice. More often than not the seltzers are also lower alcohol than cocktails in a can or wine.

SWAPS

Cocktail cans (10g+ of sugar) → Hard seltzer (2g sugar)
Less alcohol, less sugar and the same fun at a party.

Gin

A standard gin and tonic sounds simple, but tonic water is a sneaky sugar source. A small 200 ml bottle of regular tonic can pack around 16g of sugar, or about four teaspoons – nearly as much as a can of cola! That means a classic G&T isn't as innocent as it looks. The smarter move? Ask for gin with a low-sugar tonic. Many brands now offer 'light' or diet tonic that uses little to no sugar, often replacing it with natural sweeteners.

SWAPS

G&T with full-sugar tonic (16g sugar) → G&T with diet tonic (1-2g)
Cut sugar by 90%.

Cocktails

Many cocktails rely on sugar syrup for flavour, making them no better than dessert in disguise. A margarita, for instance, often contains sugary syrup or sweet liqueur and can easily deliver dozens of grams of sugar in one glass. Instead, opt for drinks that get their flavour from herbs, bitters, or fresh ingredients without added sugar. Think along the lines of a martini or a whisky on the rocks. Your taste buds might miss the super-sweet hit at first, but they'll adjust – and your body will thank you.

SWAPS

Margarita (12g sugar) → Vodka soda with lime (0g sugar)
Keep the ritual, ditch the sugar bomb.

THE FREEZER SECTION

Now it's time to get a little chilly and immerse ourselves in the rather unloved, unsexy section of the supermarket, where most of us reluctantly go to find frozen chips, pizzas and ice cream. But, with a few clever swaps tucked under your arm, you can turn the freezer aisles into a cornucopia of surprisingly inexpensive nutrition.

In 1922, it was one Clarence Birdseye who invented the process of flash-freezing foods to seal in goodness. That's the same Captain Birdseye you'll know from your packet of fish fingers. Well, he probably didn't have a white beard and a wry smile, but he's important! Birdseye's invention locked in freshness fast and so changed the way the world ate.

Freezers only started appearing in UK supermarkets in the 1950s. By the 1980s, frozen peas, fish fingers, and ready meals had become household staples. Frozen food was marketed as futuristic convenience back then, but today it's often dismissed as second-rate.

I'm going to change your view on that. Because frozen fruit and vegetables often hold *more* nutrients than fresh and can be up to 40% cheaper, because it is so much easier to manage supply chains and reduce wastage.

THE GOOD
Fruit and veg – frozen at peak ripeness, plus
wild-caught fish fillets.

THE BAD
Super-cheap, low-quality breaded nuggets that need deep frying, deep pan pizzas, ready meals, potato products and frozen desserts.

THE HEALTHY
The good news about the freezer section is on average you will find less preservatives added because freezing does that for us. So the frozen burgers, and the odd fish finger will likely be better for you than the chilled version.

Fabulously frozen fruit and vegetables

Forget everything you remember about soggy cauliflower and fat floury peas and have a rummage in those freezers. Frozen produce is picked at peak ripeness, when it's most nutrient-dense, and then flash-frozen within hours of picking. This process effectively pauses the degradation of the vitamins, minerals and antioxidants, preserving the nutritional value until you're ready to eat.

Freezing produce also locks in nutrients that might otherwise be lost during transportation and storage. And here's the real winner: frozen fruits and vegetables are often more affordable than their fresh counterparts.

Let's break down the price comparisons:

- Blueberries – over 40% saving
- Broccoli – over 45% saving
- Spinach – over 65% saving

Now, I know what you're going to say. Frozen doesn't always taste as good as fresh. And I'd agree with you, but there are simple ways to make these changes more palatable for your taste buds too. For fruit, use them in smoothies and you won't notice the difference. For your morning yoghurt, make blueberries into a simple compote and they'll taste just as delicious. When you've got a bag of frozen spinach you can add some to many meals to boost the vegetable intake without anyone noticing. With broccoli, steam instead of boil to avoid it going mushy. Or even better still, roast frozen veg in the oven for a nice crunch.

Don't let the health halo of fresh produce blind you to the benefits of frozen. By topping up with frozen, you can enjoy better nutrient retention, amazing cost savings, and reduce food waste. Around half of all global food emissions come from food waste.[40] The average UK household wastes about £470 worth of food each year and a large portion of that is fresh fruits and veggies that have gone bad before being eaten. Frozen produce not only locks in nutrients but also extends shelf life, meaning you only cook what you need.

If your children say they don't like peas, try them on petit pois (smaller, sweeter little green bursts of flavour on a plate) and mix in sweetcorn kernels to boost their vegetable intake. Rummage around in those freezers and you'll find sliced or diced onions, sliced frozen peppers and mushrooms, chopped garlic, brussels sprouts, sweet potato chunks, ready-chopped casserole vegetables and Mediterranean-style roasting vegetables too.

Something fishy

Most supermarket freezers are groaning with breaded and battered fish in an assortment of shapes and sizes, and frozen UPF convenience foods packed with oil and additives. It's not an ideal way to stay healthy. But there are some great swaps to try and frozen fish is one of my favourites.

I know the idea of 'fresh' fish always seems more appealing, but the reality is very different. Most fish is frozen at source as it spoils quickly, which means the fresh fish you are buying is often defrosted fish. Why not just buy frozen and defrost it yourself?

Fewer preservatives

Another great thing about frozen foods is they don't need to be packed with preservatives, which is great news. For example, bagged croissants you pick up in the bread aisle will often contain emulsifiers (mono- and di-glycerides of fatty acids) to help extend their shelf life. But you'll find a healthier additive-free croissant in the freezer section which you can pop into the oven to bake 'as fresh' at home.

Check the packaging on any fresh beef burgers and you're likely to find preservatives such as sodium meta-bisulphite to help extend quality on the shelf, but frozen quarter pounders don't need so many chemical additives because the freezing process does the job for them.

Now let's break down the swaps.

SWAPS

Fresh blueberries → Frozen blueberries
40% cheaper, same antioxidants.

Fresh spinach → Frozen spinach
65% cheaper, just as nutritious.

Broccoli → Frozen broccoli
45% cheaper, no waste.

'Fresh' fish (defrosted) → Frozen fish
Same product, lower cost, longer shelf life.

**Fresh croissants (with emulsifiers) →
Frozen bake-at-home croissants**
Fewer additives, healthier ingredients, and fresher
taste straight from your oven.

**Fresh burgers (with preservatives) →
Frozen quarter pounders**
Freezing removes the need for sodium
metabisulphite, keeping the ingredients cleaner.

**Frozen breaded fish/chicken →
Non-breaded wild fish**
Ditch the oil and filler, keep the protein.

Can I have an ice lolly?

If you've got children or grandchildren, you'll be familiar with the cries of, 'I want an ice lolly, can I have an ice lolly, pleeeeaase!' Those little puppy-dog eyes and appealing smiles as they beg us for a frozen treat – how can we resist? I know I can't, and I don't think we should be denying our children little moments of pleasure. Plus (bonus) it may well give us an extra five or ten minutes of peace and quiet!

The funny part about this constant summer battle is that the first ice lolly was actually invented by an 11-year-old kid in 1905. Frank Epperson left a glass of soda with a stirring stick in it outside overnight. It froze, and kickstarted a century of parents battling demands for frozen lollies.

Inevitably, when you're leaning over the freezer trying to work out which lollies to buy, you'll face good, bad and healthy options. The key to making a healthy choice is, as ever, how often you make the choice, and what you choose. It might be ok to give the kids an ice lolly every day when you're on holiday, but perhaps it should be a less frequent treat at other times. In terms of choice, you might be surprised at the healthier and equally satisfying options for your kids that you might have overlooked.

THE GOOD
A simple ingredients list with no additives and very little sugar, ideally organic lollies or even homemade yoghurt pops.

THE BAD
Oversized, high-sugar lollies packed with chemical additives that can deliver up to 73% of a child's daily sugar allowance in one hit.

THE HEALTHY
Small lollies that satisfy the craving with less sugar: dairy-based (Mini Milk, Little Jude's) offer a treat while containing only a teaspoon of sugar.

Let's break down the usual suspects – here's a quick rundown of the sugar content in some popular choices:

- **Del Monte 100% Juice 75ml:** 15g of sugar per lolly or almost 4 teaspoons.
- **Calippo Orange Mini 80ml**: 14g of sugar per lolly or 3.5 teaspoons.
- **Rowntrees Fruit Pastilles 65ml:** 11.5g of sugar per lolly or almost 3 teaspoons.
- **Fab 58ml:** 10g of sugar per lolly or 2.5 teaspoons.
- **Twister Mini 50ml**: 8.6g of sugar per lolly or just over 2 teaspoons.
- **Mini Milk 35ml** – 4.1g sugar per lolly or just one teaspoon.
- **Little Jude's 35ml** – 2.7g of sugar per lolly.

(Note: you may be surprised to see a 100% juice lolly at the top of the sugar list, but fruit juice is still classed as a free sugar and acts in the body the same way as an added sugar.)

Now, I get it, it's a treat – but the sugar impact can add up. An 80% drop in your sugar per lolly means you cut out three teaspoons of sugar, which is a huge opportunity to stop your kids from overdosing on the sweet stuff. If you have one lolly a day for 30 days of ice-lolly weather (I'm being optimistic here!), you'll be rescuing them from over 90 teaspoons of sugar over the summer.

Sugar content will vary according to the size of the lolly, but portion control matters. Most of us will eat whatever is put in front of us. In fact, you might be surprised how little you need to hit that sweet-tooth craving. Over time, choosing smaller, lower-sugar options will help to shape healthier taste buds, so your children grow up less dependent on excessive sweetness. Ice lollies can still be fun and refreshing, but when you buy them mini-sized and milk-based, they shift from being a sugar bomb to a balanced treat.

SWAPS

Big lollies → Mini lollies
Smaller portions still hit the sweet spot but keep kids well below daily sugar limits.

Del Monte 100% Juice Lolly (15g sugar) → Twister Mini (8.6g sugar)
Half the sugar; juice still counts as free sugar.

Calippo (14g sugar) → Mini Milk (4.1g sugar)
Almost 75% less sugar.

Mini Milk → Frozen yoghurt pops
These are a lifesaver for a teething baby or a hot summer afternoon. Take plain Greek yoghurt, mix in some berries and a squeeze of lemon, and pour into ice lolly moulds. Freeze for a few hours. You get creamy, tangy frozen yoghurt ice cream that is packed with nutrients and far lower in sugar than shop-bought ice lollies.

How much sugar is too much?
According to NHS advice:

- Adults should have no more than 30g of free sugars a day (7 teaspoons).
- Children aged 7 to 10 should have no more than 24g of free sugars a day (6 teaspoons).
- Children aged 4 to 6 should have no more than 19g of free sugars a day (4.75 teaspoons).

Considering the above guidelines, one Calippo provides 73% of your kid's (4-6 years) daily sugar intake or 58% if your child is aged seven or older. With just one of these lollies, you're consuming a significant chunk of your daily sugar allowance, so it's worth considering your choices and choosing a healthier option.

That's why I'm such a fan of making the lolly switch for my kids. It's a powerful step towards healthier eating for your little ones without having to face the argument or tantrum if you say an outright 'no'. So, next time you're reaching into the freezer, remember that not all ice lollies are created equal.

KIDS' SWAPS

LUNCHBOXES

It's 7:00am on a weekday and the lunchbox scramble begins. You're juggling breakfast, tracking down homework and sports kit, and trying to pack something that your child will actually eat at school. When you're rushing, it's tempting to hit autopilot – a ham sandwich, a packet of crisps, maybe a flavoured yoghurt or drink. Sound familiar? Busy parents often fall back on the same lunch routine because it's quick and battle-tested when you're dealing with fussy eaters. Believe me, I know! But those convenient foods are filling little tummies with more sugar and processed ingredients than you realise, and that's going to send your child on a roller coaster of blood sugar spikes and dips, which will make it harder for them to focus in class. Additives and UPF ingredients they contain have been linked to behavioural issues like hyperactivity. Over time, relying on them too often can also crowd out the nutrient-rich foods that kids need to support steady growth and brain development.

The good news is that, with a few simple swaps and a dash of planning, you can turn that midday meal into a mini-health boost for your child. Let's unpack how to upgrade the classic kids' lunchbox in simple, practical and totally doable ways.

THE GOOD
Sourdough sandwiches with slices of real chicken,
cheese, or hummus; crunchy veg sticks; Greek yoghurt
with fruit; water or diluted juices.

THE BAD
Ham sandwiches made with ultra-processed slices,
crisps, chocolate, biscuits, and juice cartons – all
high in UPFs, sugar, salt and additives, and low in
real nutrients.

THE HEALTHY
Cheese sandwiches (ideally wholemeal bread),
chicken wraps, plain yoghurts, fresh fruit. Familiar
but with some nutritional value.

Beware the UPF lunchbox

The ham sandwich is a British lunchbox legend. In fact, surveys show that a sandwich is the main component of most packed lunches and ham is the number one filling choice for kids (57%).[41] There's a comforting familiarity in that perfect combo of soft bread and salty ham. It might be popular, but it deserves a closer look.

For a start, not all ham is ham. The cheap processed ham slices found in many lunchboxes are often pumped up with water, preservatives and fillers – some packaged ham is as little as 60-70% meat, with the rest being water, salt, sugar, stabilisers and preservatives. It might look like the real deal, but in fact is more likely to be a reconstituted meat product loaded with extras your child's body doesn't need. If the idea of paying for watered-down ham isn't enough to give you pause, consider this: health experts have long flagged processed meats such as ham as something we should only eat occasionally. The World Health Organization classifies processed meat as carcinogenic to humans – meaning there's strong evidence it can increase cancer risk over time.[42]

This doesn't mean a single ham sandwich will doom your child's health. Context is key. If ham sandwiches are sneaking into that lunchbox every day, the bad stuff starts to add up. Most sliced ham you buy in the supermarket counts as a UPF. Crisps? UPF. Flavoured yoghurt? UPF. We know repeated exposure to all those additives and preservatives can have long-term effects, particularly on our children.

UK diet studies have revealed some shocking findings that even I struggle to believe. One of the most recent shows that 82% of calories in packed lunches come from UPFs.[43] That crowding out of fresh, whole foods can contribute to everything from higher obesity rates to deficiencies in important nutrients. So, reducing processed items in the lunchbox – even just a bit – can make a meaningful difference.

Healthier lunchbox upgrades

Parents need solutions, not just warnings. So, let's swap out the usual lunchbox staples for better options that are nutritious, yummy, not too expensive and realistic for busy families (i.e. your kids might actually enjoy them!). Below is a quick-glance table of typical lunchbox items and some clever alternatives. These swaps emphasise whole or minimally processed foods that pack in nutrients and cut back on added junk. Even small changes – such as choosing a different snack each day or switching up the drink – will add up to big health gains over a school year!

Lunchbox item	Smart swap	Why it's better
Processed ham on white bread	Cheese or chicken sandwich on sourdough	Real cheese or unprocessed chicken provides protein and calcium without artificial additives. Sourdough bread adds fibre and steady energy.
Crisps	Cheesies or rice/lentil cakes	These still satisfy the crunch craving but with healthier ingredients. Rice cakes deliver fibre without the excess fried fat.
Chocolate or dried fruit gummies	Dark chocolate 85%+ or fresh fruit.	Real fruit gives natural sweetness plus vitamins and fibre. Dark chocolate is high in polyphenols and so low in sugar that a couple of squares can be enjoyed daily.
Flavoured yoghurt	Greek yoghurt with mix-ins	Greek yoghurt has zero added sugar and triples the protein of normal flavoured kiddie yoghurts, supporting strong bones and steady energy. Topping it with fruit and seeds adds fibre and vitamins.

Lunchbox item	Smart swap	Why it's better
Fruit juice box/sugary drink	Water or no-added-sugar drinks	Hydration without the sugar overload. Water is best for teeth and overall health. If your child wants juice, I'll share some recommendations in this chapter for pouches that give that fruity taste without the artificial ingredients or sugar rush. Fewer empty calories mean better concentration and energy levels through the afternoon.

Swapping in just one or two of these alternatives can make a big difference, because if it happens every day the compound effect can be massive. You'll be cutting down on ultra-processed extras and adding more wholesome fuel. The goal is familiar foods with a healthier twist. Get creative! Depending on your child, you might need a little bit of trial and error, but most kids love cheese, fruit and yoghurt. With one or two swaps, they'll still get to enjoy a crunchy snack and a treat, but you can be confident that you're giving them better versions of their old favourites. In many cases, they might not even realise anything has changed – but they will certainly feel satisfied and ener-gised, rather than riding a sugar high at lunchtime.

Cunning lunchbox hacks

Even with better food choices, mornings can be hectic. How can you streamline healthy lunch prep for your kids when you're half-awake and pressed for time? Try these practical lunchbox hacks that will save your sanity and boost your little one's health factor:

- **Plan for leftovers:** Every so often, you can leverage dinner to lighten the lunch load by cooking an extra portion and setting it aside for the next day's lunchbox. Roast chicken or beef on Sunday? Slice the leftovers for sandwiches or wraps on Monday instead of reaching for processed deli ham. Even an extra meatball can be reinvented as a filling in a wholemeal wrap with lettuce and a bit of cheese the next day. This cook-once, eat-twice approach means the lunch protein is a real, home-cooked food and you will have saved time (and money).

- **Batch and prep**: On a quiet evening or at the weekend, prep a few grab-and-pack items. For example, wash and cut carrot, cucumber, or pepper sticks and store them in the fridge in a container of water to stay crisp. Bake a batch of healthy egg muffins and freeze them. You can pull one out in the morning, and it will thaw by lunch. Having these ready-to-go sides and snacks makes lunchbox assembly just a little easier on chaotic mornings.

SWAPS

**Ham sandwich (processed slices) → Chicken
or cheese sandwich**
Less processing, same protein.

White bread → Wholemeal or sourdough
More fibre, better energy release.

**Crisps → Rice cakes, Cheesies or
mini cheese portions**
Reduce fried oils, add protein or fibre.

**Chocolate bar → Fresh fruit or 85% dark
chocolate squares**
Swap sugar spikes for antioxidants and vitamins.

Flavoured yoghurt → Greek yoghurt with fruit and seeds
Triple the protein, skip the added sugar.

Fruit juice carton → Water or lower-sugar diluted juice
Hydration without the hidden sugar load.

Finally, remember that perfection isn't the goal. It's absolutely fine for kids to have the odd treat. The idea here is to tip the balance in favour of healthier choices on most days if you can. By avoiding the everyday ultra-processed staples and making whole or low-processed foods the norm, you will be doing wonders for your child's long-term well-being. Each healthy swap is an opportunity to pack in nutrients that support your child's growth and learning, because consistent good nutrition helps stabilise their mood and concentration in class too.

The lunchbox is such an influential part of their day. Childhood is also when taste preferences and eating habits are formed. If a child grows up thinking a ham sandwich, crisps, and a chocolate bar is a normal lunch every day, that habit may carry into adulthood. On the flip side, if they become accustomed to sourdough cheese and lettuce sandwiches as regular parts of lunch, those foods become their normal.

In the end, remember that consistency matters more than any single lunch. If most days you can include a few fresh, minimally processed items and ease back on the packaged foods, you're doing a fantastic job. And if on some crazy mornings you do end up tossing in a biscuit – it's ok. Parenting is hard enough; lunch doesn't need to be perfect, just a bit better where possible.

One way to make this easier is to start shifting taste preferences at home. For example, if you gradually introduce kids to darker chocolate, it helps normalise those flavours so they're less likely to reject healthier options in their lunchbox at school. Take it slow; milk to normal dark chocolate, then 70% and eventually 85% makes a difference. To make it easier to get creative with their lunchbox, make sure you have the right tools. Keep a few small pots for their lunchbox handy so you can spoon in Greek yoghurt with berries, portion out some nuts, or pack sliced veggies.

Beware the mini juice carton

Juice cartons are a super-convenient staple of school lunches or a day out at the park. A healthy alternative to squash or fizzy pop, right? Wrong! Fruit juice might contain a few nutrients and none of the additives you find in a UPF drink, but it's packed with quick-release sugar. A mini 200ml box of apple juice contains 22g sugar – that's a child's full daily allowance in one hit.

It doesn't matter whether I take the kids to the beach,

the zoo or for a local walk that ends up at a café, my three-year-old will catch sight of the fridge stocked with cute little cartons and say 'Appy!' (apple juice). Those fruit characters peering back at him promise pure sugary bliss. Yes, I do give in to him sometimes. I don't want him to miss out on the joys of going to a café and it gives me and my wife the chance to enjoy a coffee in peace. But it frustrates me that the food industry create this parental battle for us. Why can't they just make lower-sugar options?

Well, the good news is that they can and that they are starting to change. Choosing the right one could be the difference between a sugar spike and a healthier, happier kid. Let's unpack the kids' juice jungle.

THE GOOD
Water as the daily go-to, with juice cartons saved for an occasional treat.

THE BAD
Standard fruit juice cartons (200ml apple juice = 22g sugar) or 'no added sugar' cartons which contain artificial sweeteners – less sugar, but a horrible cocktail of chemical additives.

THE HEALTHY
Diluted juices or 'nothing artificial' cartons with reduced sugar, such as Capri-Sun Nothing Artificial (8.8g sugar per 100ml). When choosing juice, go for the lowest-sugar diluted options with no artificial additives.

We know too much sugar isn't good for our kids. The NHS recommends children aged 4-6 should have no more than 19g of sugar a day, and those aged 7-10 should have no more than 24g per day. But a standard apple juice carton (200ml) contains over five teaspoons of sugar. It might look like the healthier option at a glance – it's just fruit juice after all! That's natural fruit sugar. But take any form of sugar delivered in those concentrated doses, without the fibre protection provided by the whole fruit, and you get a one-way ticket to Sugarville. And for those of you who are screaming, 'but Innocent smoothies are ok? right? right?' The theory goes that because it's a smoothie there is more fibre in there. But the truth is that in 100g of apple you'd expect 2.4g of fibre, yet in 100ml of Innocent apple smoothie we only see 0.6g of fibre. That's 75% less than whole fruit and not enough to protect your little one from the 4-5 teaspoons of natural free sugar they are about to receive.

The alternative? You might be tempted to reach for juice cartons labelled 'no added sugar' or 'sugar-free', but here's where we hit another issue. These options contain the same artificial sweeteners as diet soft drinks, which introduce their own set of concerns. Studies show they can affect taste preferences and disrupt gut health – and they're certainly not the golden ticket to healthy hydration we might hope for. Just recently, the BBC published a report from the Scientific Advisory Committee on Nutrition (SACN) recommending that younger children should not be given ANY drinks containing artificial sweeteners, and this includes sugar-free squash.[44]

Thankfully, it looks like the industry is beginning to clean up its act. You can now buy juices with lower natural sugar content, diluted with water to keep the sweetness in check without resorting to additives. Look out for brands like Cawston Press and Ninju, which are leading the way in reducing the sugar content of kids' juices. Ninju has achieved a massive 50% reduction.

So, I look for juice cartons that strike a balance and aim for them to be an occasional treat on weekends rather than a daily lunchbox staple. Children should fundamentally learn to drink water and, sorry to say it, but this is the hard part of parenting where we need to take accountability and lead by example as the adult. If we go out as a family, it's water 90% of the time for me – alongside a coffee of course. Kids do as they see, not as we say.

By choosing these options you'll be fostering healthier habits by helping to train your children's taste buds to crave less sugar. Another good option I've discovered on my many journeys down the supermarket aisles is, believe it or not, Capri-Sun. They have a 'nothing artificial' range that is just 10% juice and a little bit of natural sweetness from a plant-based sweetener called stevia. That makes a 200ml pouch contain 8.8g of sugar, still two teaspoons of sugar per pouch, but a good saving of 41% sugar in their juice intake compared to an Innocent smoothie.

SWAPS

**Apple juice carton (20g sugar per 200ml) →
Diluted juice drink (8-10g sugar)**
Half the sugar with the same fruity hit.

**'No Added Sugar' Fruit Shoot (with artificial sweeteners)
→ Low-sugar natural juice**
Cleaner ingredients that avoid the artificial sweeteners trap.

> **Innocent smoothie (150ml, 15-17g sugar) →**
> **Capri-Sun Nothing Artificial (200ml, 8.8g sugar)**
> 41% sugar saving and much cheaper in the long run.

The good news for your purse is this range of Capri-Sun costs around half the price of smoothies per 100ml (at the time of writing). So, by simply switching from Innocent to Capri-Sun Nothing Artificial, you can save money and reduce your kids' sugar intake by 41%, which equates to 2.2kg of sugar savings per year. Health doesn't always have to be more expensive.

Of course, there's one important exception to the rule worth noting. For children living with type 1 diabetes, drinks like apple juice can be an essential part of managing a hypo because the quick release of sugar helps raise blood glucose levels rapidly – precisely the reason they aren't ideal as an everyday drink for everyone else.

SNACKS

It's 3pm. Schools out, and the snack attack begins. Your kids walk through the door starving and it's hours until their evening meal, or you've got to find something to keep them fuelled through after-school clubs. It's so easy to reach for the usual suspects – crisps, biscuits, chocolate bars, or flavoured yoghurt. But these typical kids' snacks are often packed with sugar and low in nutrients, which sets our little ones up for those notorious energy spikes and crashes, bad teeth and poor health. In the UK, children are consuming astonishing amounts of sugar and the data according to Public Health England shows that 4 to 10 year-olds put away close to 5,000 sugar cubes per year or over 20kg on average. That's roughly three times the recommended maximum! Official NHS guidelines advise that children aged 4 to 6 should have no more than 19g of free sugars a day (about five sugar cubes), and 7 to 10-year-olds no more than 24g. Yet a single chocolate bar can contain more than six cubes of sugar (over 20g), which is a young child's daily limit in one hit.

Bossing the mid-afternoon snack attack

Kids' snacks need to help build bodies, not just fill stomachs, and many popular snacks contribute virtually no fibre, protein, or vitamins to the nutritional mix. It is no surprise, then, that children whose diets are heavy in these ultra-processed snack foods end up with health and behavioural issues. The good news? By simply swapping out the worst offenders for better options, you can take big steps towards boosting your children's health without the risk of tantrums.

THE GOOD
Greek yoghurt with fruit, mini cheeses (Babybel, Cheesies), homemade trail mix (seeds and coconut flakes), which combine protein, fibre, and healthy fats to support steady energy and growth.

THE BAD
Crisps, biscuits, chocolate bars. I'm sorry but these just shouldn't be daily staples for kids.

THE HEALTHY
Rice cakes, plain digestive biscuits, flavoured yoghurts are familiar and convenient, with more nutrients and less sugar than conventional choices.

Healthy snacking for kids isn't about perfection or banning fun foods; it's about finding smarter swaps that kids will actually eat without them realising it is healthy for them. Here are some parent-approved swap ideas to consider:

SWAPS

Crisps → Cheesies

A small bag of crisps is basically fried starch, plus salt and a heap of artificial additives sprinkled on top. By contrast, Cheesies are small slices of 100% cheese, which are baked till crunchy. For about 120 calories per pack and no sugar at all, you get a cheesy, salty crunch with the added benefit of protein and calcium from real cheese. You'll find them in larger supermarkets and health food stores such as Holland & Barrett. Another option is mini cheese portions such as Babybel (4g of protein, 0g sugar, and important nutrients for about 30-40p a piece.)

Chocolate bars → Nut-based bars

Kids love the sweetness of chocolate, but a standard bar contains up to 25g of sugar. Nut-based bars such as Kind bars (if the school allows nuts) can offer protein, good fats and fibre alongside a lot less sweetness (4-8g of sugar per bar or 16% sugar). The goal is a treat that won't send your child bouncing off the walls.

Flavoured yoghurt → Greek yoghurt with fruit

yoghurt pots and pouches are a better choice than crisps or chocolate, but they still typically add unnecessary sugar, flavourings and additives. For example, a little pot of Munch Bunch contains 10.7g of total sugars per 100g, which is more than double that of plain yoghurt.
By swapping to plain Greek yoghurt, you get zero added sugar (just the natural lactose, about 3-4g per 100g) and roughly triple the protein, which will help your child feel fuller for longer. Add a handful of blueberries or chopped strawberries and you have a delicious, naturally sweet snack with fibre and nutrients.

Biscuits → Rice cakes

Many biscuits are loaded with sugar (30-35% sugar for the average chocolate chip cookie), but if you fancy a 50% sugar saving, all you have to do is switch to plain digestives at about 15% sugar. A rice cake, however, can give that same crunchy moment without any sugar. Top it with a little peanut butter and a few banana slices and you are good to go. Two lightly topped rice cakes can satisfy the munchies at a fraction of the sugar. You'll also find those mini rice cakes marketed for toddlers, which are portioned and come in fruity flavours. They have a low sugar content of around 7.8% (from added apple juice). Watch out for the adults' flavoured rice cake as they can be up to 20% sugar; the ones coated in chocolate are surprisingly high in sugar too at 32%.

Of course, children always care more about taste and fun than what's on the nutritional labels, but the key is finding options they'll genuinely enjoy. Many of the swaps above still feel like treats – they're just *better-for-you* treats.

Homemade snacks

Store-bought solutions are convenient, but some of the best kids' snacks come straight from your kitchen – you can often whip them up in just minutes, using very basic ingredients. Making snacks at home means you control exactly what goes into them, and it can save money too. Here are a couple of DIY snack ideas that I swear by as a busy parent:

- **Homemade trail mix:** Shop-bought trail mixes can be expensive and are often loaded with more raisins than nuts or chocolate. Making your own is cheaper and can be tailored to your child's taste. Combine unsalted peanuts or cashews, some pumpkin or sunflower seeds, a few chopped dried apricots (the lowest sugar dried fruit) and maybe a couple of dark chocolate chips or some popcorn. Portion it into little containers or mini zip bags. This trail mix provides a great balance of protein, healthy fats, and a touch of sweetness.

- **Fruit reinvented:** Often, presentation is half the battle with kids – a plain apple might be boring, but apple slices arranged like smiley faces with a quick dollop of peanut butter can be much more exciting. Create fruit kebabs on cocktail sticks, alternating pieces of apple with berries and cheese cubes. Freezing a slice of watermelon and grating it into a bowl makes delicious shaved ice. These ideas take just a few minutes and turn everyday produce into treat-like experiences. Do be mindful of choking hazards with younger kids: foods like whole nuts, whole grapes, or hard crudités can be dangerous for under-fives. Always adapt textures (e.g. ground nuts on yoghurt instead of whole, halved grapes, softer steamed veggie sticks for toddlers). Healthy snacks are only good if they're also safe.

SWAPS

Crisps → Cheesies or Babybel
From fried starch to real protein and calcium.

**Chocolate bar (25g sugar) → Nut-based
bar (4-8g sugar)**
Half or quarter the sugar, added fibre and healthy fats.

**Flavoured yoghurts (10.7g sugar/100g) → Plain
Greek yoghurt with fruit**
(3-4g natural sugar/100g) – triple the protein,
no added sugar.

**Chocolate chip cookies (30-35% sugar) →
Plain digestives (15% sugar)**
50% less sugar for the same crunch.

Digestives → Rice cakes with peanut butter and banana
Keep the crunch, add fibre and protein.

Why kids' snacks matter

Making a little effort to optimise your snack selection is even more important for kids than for adults because children are growing fast, building bones, muscles and brains at a rapid rate. They require a steady supply of protein, healthy fats, vitamins and minerals to do so. Each snack is a chance to provide those building blocks. A sugar-laden snack gives essentially nothing beneficial (aside from quick energy), whereas a nutrient-dense one such as yoghurt, cheese, or fruit provides raw materials for growth. Think of every healthy snack as an investment in your child's growing body and, importantly, their long-term eating habits too. Childhood is when taste preferences and eating habits are formed. So, if cookies and crisps are their norm, this sets a precedent they may carry into adulthood. On the flip side, if your children get used to eating carrot sticks with hummus or apple slices with peanut butter, they're more likely to continue those habits later.

Many adults today struggle with sugar cravings largely because we grew up with so many sweet snacks. Just think back to those childhood favourites that still give you nostalgia pangs today. When you're offering your children snacks you have a chance to break that cycle. By making healthy snacks the default, you'll be teaching your children that treats are occasional, and real food is the go-to. As they grow, they'll thank you later, maybe not in words, but in strong healthy bodies and sound eating habits.

Lastly, let's acknowledge reality – no parent is perfect, even me! Striving to deliver for 100% healthy snacks 24/7 is unrealistic. Birthdays, holidays, or just exhausting days will happen, and sometimes a chocolate biscuit hits the spot. That's ok! What matters is the overall pattern. Health isn't about being perfect, it's just about making the next choice a little bit better. Every swap, every slightly better choice, adds up and it means you'll be stacking the odds in your child's favour.

PERSONAL
CARE
SWAPS

SHAMPOO AND SUNCREAM

Every morning, millions of us perform a well-rehearsed routine: brush teeth, lather up in the shower, apply deodorant. Maybe you smear on a bit of body lotion, or suncream for good measure. After all, personal hygiene is all about keeping clean teeth, a clean body, and protecting your skin against the ravages of age.

As you wander down the supermarket aisles you might grab a pack of deodorants on special offer, pick up the toothpaste the kids like the taste of, or grab a shampoo because it smells good or it promises luscious locks.

But what if I told you some of these personal care products could be doing you more harm than good?

The personal care and beauty sector today contributes over £27 billion to the UK economy, and what has all that innovation and chemistry advancements led us to? Are we cleaner than ever? Or are we unknowingly dousing ourselves in harmful chemicals? In this chapter, we'll squeeze out the truth about some of the most common bathroom staples: toothpaste, deodorant, shampoo and suncream.

Let's all lather up

The shampoo aisle is home to a variety of bubbly lathers and a chemical alphabet soup. It's no secret that most shampoos contain surfactants such as sodium lauryl sulfate (SLS), or its milder cousin sodium laureth sulfate, to provide that satisfying foamy cleanse. Many also contain parabens added as preservatives to prevent mould and bacteria. If you've ever read the ingredients list on the back of a shampoo bottle and felt a stab of anxiety, you're not alone.

There's no doubt that SLS is a strong cleanser – it's very effective at cutting grease, which is why it's also used in washing-up liquid. But because it's such a good degreaser, SLS can strip the scalp of its natural oils. At high concentrations or with prolonged skin contact, SLS can irritate skin or scalp and cause dryness and itching. It can certainly worsen dandruff and scalp issues if you have them, in part because the scalp is often more susceptible to absorption than other areas of skin, due to its high density of hair follicles.

Studies show that when SLS is applied to skin, a small amount of the chemical might penetrate. However, any that does enter the body is swiftly dealt with by your liver and kidneys, which break SLS down and flush it out within a day. So absorption isn't the worry. The real downside is that it can be too drying or irritating for some people's skin if they're sensitive. The British Journal of Dermatology states, 'All patient groups showed a higher degree of skin-barrier disruption and inflammation than did controls in response to SLS.' Many UK brands now offer sulphate-free shampoos instead, which are a better option if you have sensitive skin.

Another very common ingredient added to shampoos, lotions, makeup and more is parabens (such as methylparaben and propylparaben), which are added as a preservative. Some parabens share structural similarities to hormones, which means, if absorbed through the skin, they can disrupt the body's natural hormone balance. Parabens also have a weak oestrogenic-like effect in the body, meaning they can bind to oestrogen receptors.

Parabens can be absorbed through skin and studies have found measurable paraben levels in the urine of pretty much everyone these days, showing how common our exposure is. But absorbed does not automatically equal dangerous.[45] The concentration matters. So far, no direct causal link between paraben exposure from cosmetics and any major illness has been proven. The amounts we absorb from shampoos or lotions are very small, and our bodies also break parabens down and excrete them relatively quickly. In fact, the EU strictly regulates the maximum concentration allowed in products sold in the UK. In recent years, many parabens have been banned as a precaution, leaving only the safer, shorter-chain parabens in use.

Despite these precautions, there is an ongoing debate about cumulative exposure. If you think about it, a typical adult might use shampoo, conditioner, body wash, moisturiser, suncream, and makeup every day. One 2020 review did caution that while a single paraben-containing cosmetic isn't a health hazard, using a lot of such products together could, in theory, push exposure into a zone of concern.[46] Natalia Matwiejczuk, in the *Journal of Toxicology* puts it this way: 'excessive quantities of cosmetic preparations containing these compounds may lead to the development of unfavourable health outcomes.' As a practical step, the review's authors advised trying to avoid simultaneous use of many paraben-containing items. This doesn't mean you're doomed if you love one shampoo that has parabens, but swapping a couple of products to paraben-free versions could reduce your overall exposure. Many brands now make paraben-free formulas (such as Green People, Aveda, The Body Shop, Palmers and Moroccanoil) – you'll see this especially in products aimed at babies too.

One more common chemical ingredient worth a quick mention: phthalates. These are added to many products as fragrance fixatives (to make the scents last longer), or as solvents dissolving and dispersing ingredients to improve product texture and spreadability. These aren't usually called out specifically on the product label, but they can be hiding under the term 'fragrance' or listed as 'parfum' on labels. They've been flagged as potential endocrine disruptors too, which interfere with the body's hormones. The considerations are similar to parabens – the evidence of harm at cosmetic exposure levels is inconclusive, but consumers may choose to avoid them as a precaution. Thankfully, the industry is increasingly moving away from using these, with more zero-fragrance products cropping up in the market to provide alternatives.

SWAPS

Ordinary shampoo → Sulphate-free shampoo
Gentler on scalp, still effective cleansing.

> **Ordinary shampoo, body wash and lotion →**
> **Paraben-free shampoo, body wash and lotion**
>
> **Fragranced products (which may contain phthalates) →**
> **Fragrance-free products**
> Cut hidden endocrine disruptors.

Putting suncreams in the shade

If there's one thing the British summer teaches us, it's to be ready when the sun finally decides to make an appearance. And when it does, out comes the suncream. But like everything we put on our skin, suncream deserves a closer look.

Let's start with the clear benefits. Suncream protects us from the sun's ultraviolet (UV) rays – UVA, which ages the skin, and UVB, which burns it. And let's be clear upfront, burning our skin in a long tanning session is not and has never been a good idea. The NHS and Cancer Research UK recommend using suncream with at least SPF 30 to reduce your risk of melanoma and other skin cancers.[47] For the UK, where rates of melanoma have more than doubled since the early 1990s, this is a really big topic we need to address. Have we increased our sun exposure by double since the 1990s? Are we all working outside increasingly? Or is something else at play? Now to put this into perspective, when you look at Europe, the highest rates of skin cancer don't seem to be in the countries with the most sun – the top three are Denmark, Holland and Sweden.[48]

Dermatologist Richard Weller is quoted in the *Journal*

of Investigative Dermatology as saying, 'We need to stand back and take a more holistic view of UV exposure and human health.'[49] Multiple strands of evidence also point to the importance of sunlight on health and, if you reverse it, you see all-cause mortality is markedly higher in winter than in summer.

Most suncreams use ingredients such as oxybenzone, octinoxate, avobenzone, and octocrylene, which absorb UV rays and convert them into heat, which is then released from the skin. They undergo a chemical reaction with UV radiation to prevent it from damaging skin cells.

Several of the ingredients found in chemical suncreams have come under scrutiny in recent years:

- Oxybenzone has been linked to hormone disruption in studies.[50] The author states Oxybenzone has 'endocrine disrupting properties, endorsing recent European regulatory efforts to limit human exposure.'
- In 2024, the European Commission found it could not determine the safety of current octinoxate use levels due to concerns about endocrine disruption and genotoxicity.[51]

Both oxybenzone and octinoxate have been banned in Hawaii and parts of the US due to their damaging effects on coral reefs. This raises the question: if it's unsafe for marine life, should we be smothering our kids in it?

In the face of these fears, it is good to know that the amount of these chemicals absorbed by the skin under normal use is small, and regulators, such as the EU

Scientific Committee on Consumer Safety, have deemed them safe within set limits. But, if you're using them daily for decades, that low-dose argument can begin to wear thin.

Mineral suncreams are a more natural and safer alternative because they use zinc oxide, which sits on the skin's surface and reflects UV rays like little mirrors. Mineral suncream is broad-spectrum, stable, and less likely to cause irritation, making it especially good for kids and those with sensitive skin. Some UK options include Green People, Shade, Badger, Childs Farm SPF (zinc-based), and even Boots Soltan now offers 'reef-friendly' options which remove some of the worst-offending chemicals.

SWAPS

Chemical suncream → Zinc-based mineral suncream
Fewer chemicals, safer for kids, your skin and of course the coral reefs.

Here's a simple truth: some sun exposure may be healthy and helpful to protect your skin. Think of it like a muscle that needs training in the gym; small frequent exposure and your muscle gets stronger. But if you take one trip a year to the beach and cook like a lobster, then you are asking for trouble. Covering up with clothing, wearing a hat, and seeking shade between 12pm and 2pm are all good, standard sun-safety ideas, especially for children, that should be observed. Burning isn't good, but some sun may be.

DEODRANT AND TOOTHPASTE

Next up in your personal wash bag, that trusty deodorant or antiperspirant you swipe or spray on every morning. It might seem completely harmless, but there's a small risk here that's worth learning about.

It wasn't until the 1950s, when TV advertising was introduced, that deodorant use became a daily habit for most households. Previously, frequent washing, talcum powder and herbs or scented oils had been used to keep body odour at bay. We were also more likely to wear natural linen and wool, which have antimicrobial properties that ensure odour is kept to a minimum and do not retain smell the way that modern fabrics do today.

First, a quick chemistry-of-your-armpit lesson: antiperspirants use aluminium chlorohydrate or sesquichlorohydrate as their active ingredient. These particles form little plugs in your sweat ducts, which is what keeps you dry.

Some studies have found links between aluminium exposure and neurotoxicity through various mechanisms, including oxidative stress and neuroinflammation. In the lab, aluminium can mimic oestrogen a bit (oestrogen can fuel some breast cancers) and can damage DNA in cells at high concentrations. Extensive studies have compared women who use antiperspirants vs. those who don't, and they've struggled to find a consistent link in breast cancer risk.[52] The American Cancer Institute and Cancer Research UK have both stated that there's no conclusive scientific evidence linking aluminium antiperspirants to breast cancer. However, some experts do recommend caution – Albert Moussaron et al are quoted as saying, 'In light of the precautionary principle and based on the data obtained, it is better to avoid antiperspirants that contain aluminium.'[53]

As for brain health and neurotoxicity, there is a theory that dates back decades to findings of aluminium in the plaques of Alzheimer's patients' brains, but expert consensus today is that everyday aluminium exposure is not a significant risk factor for Alzheimer's disease.[54]

What we do know is that what we put on our skin is absorbed by the body, and too much aluminium in our body can be bad for our health. Your kidneys normally do a great job flushing aluminium out. But here's where the repeated exposure, daily, for decades may not be a good idea. Imagine you are using your aluminium deodorant every day for another 50 years, but you also always love to cook your daily meals in the oven with aluminium foil. You'll be potentially increasing your aluminium consumption to higher than ideal levels. Even though this is just a theoretical concern, and no studies can truly test these compound effects, it's your body, and your choice whether you take caution here or not.

If you're keen to avoid aluminium overload, there are plenty of aluminium-free deodorants on the UK market now, such as Fussy and Wild, which use natural ingredients like coconut oil, plant extracts, and baking soda. Even big brands such as Dove now offer 0% aluminium deodorants. You might need to reapply an aluminium-free deodorant more often, especially on a hot day or if you're very active, but more large-scale, long-term studies are needed to clarify potential risks.

SWAPS

Aluminium antiperspirant → Aluminium-free deodorant
Reduce cumulative exposure.

Polishing those pearly whites

Why do we even care what's in our toothpaste, you might ask? Well, our mouths are highly absorbent and brushing our teeth for two minutes can put whatever is in that tube into our bodies and bloodstream. So, have you ever wondered what is actually in your toothpaste? Let's take a look at a typical branded toothpaste you can find everywhere:

Aqua, hydrated silica, sorbitol, glycerin, sodium lauryl sulfate, xanthan gum, aroma, titanium dioxide, PEG-6/PEG-8, sodium fluoride, sodium saccharin, carrageenan, limonene, CI 73360, CI 74160, contains: sodium fluoride 0.315% w/w (1450 ppm fluoride).

There's a lot to unpack here – and I could write chapters about some of these ingredients, but I'll try and keep it short. PEG-6 is polyethylene glycol, a derivative of petroleum. Nice. CI 73360 is Red 30, a synthetic dye produced from petroleum or coal tar sources. Yum. Then we have titanium dioxide, which was banned in the EU for use as a food additive in 2022 due to concerns about its potential toxicity, but it remains permitted in toothpaste. Not to mention the artificial sweeteners. You might now start to see why I choose a naturally derived toothpaste…

Of course, we can't talk about toothpaste without touching on fluoride. To be clear, I'm not an expert in fluoride and I can only make a judgement call for my family's health. Everyone is entitled to their own choice.

THE GOOD
Natural hydroxyapatite toothpastes: natural enamel-building.

THE BAD
Artificial toothpastes with chemicals that can be absorbed, especially by young children.

THE HEALTHY
Fluoride toothpastes without the additives: proven cavity protection.

So, what is fluoride? It's simply a naturally occurring mineral that has been found to be good for our teeth, because it makes them more resistant to attacks from plaque and sugar. In some parts of the UK, it is added to drinking water supplies and every dentist will recommend brushing your teeth with a fluoride toothpaste.

But the science of fluoride's impact on health continues to evolve, with ongoing research into the possibility of potential risks, especially during early childhood development. In high concentrations, fluoride can be bad for our health, but at the levels you find in toothpaste and tap water it is deemed safe. It's also credited with cutting rates of childhood tooth decay, and figures show a 15% increase in the number of children without dental cavities in areas with fluoridated water. Rest assured, using fluoride toothpaste in safe amounts won't cause any problems.

However, studies have shown that elevated fluoride levels can affect IQ. A meta-analysis from 2012 covering 27 cross-sectional studies on children from areas with elevated fluoride exposure found an average difference of nearly seven IQ points between children in high and low-fluoride areas.[55] The National Toxicology Program (NTP) in the US has concluded with low to moderate confidence that there is an association between higher levels of fluoride exposure and lower IQ scores in children.[56]

SWAPS

Normal chemical toothpaste → Naturally-derived toothpastes
To reduce absorption risks.

Fluoride toothpaste → Hydroxyapatite toothpastes
For natural enamel-building.

If you're uneasy or you have a toddler who loves to swallow their toothpaste, there is a simple and effective alternative in the form of toothpastes containing hydroxyapatite. This is actually the main structural component of tooth enamel and studies suggest it can help remineralise teeth.[57] Fluoride works by making your teeth more resistant to the acid formed by bacteria, which causes tooth decay. However, hydroxyapatite is a naturally occurring substance in the body and it may be more effective at remineralising enamel by filling microscopic pores in the enamel and forming a protective layer to strengthen it.

So, for me and my family, I aim for the hydroxyapatite. Now, it is a little harder to find – but you can get it in Boots and Sainsburys with brands like Gem and Parla. It is also a bit more expensive, so if you are looking to maintain your budget, just opt for a natural alternative to typical toothpastes – brands like Biomed, Kingfisher, Eco Denta are all made from natural ingredients.

Watching it all add up

One theme that ties all personal care together is cumulative exposure. A single fluoride toothpaste, one roll of a deodorant, or a few shampoo washes won't harm you and the regulators are right about that. But when you add up dozens of daily exposures across decades, the picture starts to change. A paraben in your shampoo, a phthalate in your perfume, aluminium in your deodorant, SLS in your body wash, oxybenzone in your suncream… it's the combined chemical load that worries scientists most.

The good news? Even swapping out a few staples for cleaner alternatives can meaningfully lower your exposure without making life complicated or expensive. Armed with this knowledge, you can make informed choices. Upgrade products if you want to err on the side of caution for your health, but no need to throw out everything and spend a fortune unless you want to.

SUPPLEMENTS

Aha! The vitamin aisle! This is the most fascinating part of the supermarket for me.

This aisle is really no different from any other part of the supermarket. Just look at those shelves groaning with a dizzying array of options. So many choices! There are tablets, capsules, effervescents, liquids and gummies, single supplements and combinations of all kinds in every possible shape, size, strength and form. How are you supposed to decide which vitamins to take, let alone what format to take them in?

Luckily for you, I've dedicated the last 15 years of my life to studying supplements. I've read all the books and scientific papers, and I've talked to top experts. This really would be my specialist subject if I was ever invited onto Mastermind!

In the past five years, I've worked closely with a team of nutritionists to bring out my own vitamin brand called Tonic Health, which uses the best possible combination of vitamins, minerals, and plant extracts with no added sugar, sweeteners, fillers or weird ingredients. Clearly, I'm biased and I'd love you all to pick up one of my Tonic products next time you're browsing the supermarket shelves, but it's not about me, it's about your health. So I'll try to cover all the bases, give you the knowledge I've learnt, as the supplements aisle can be a complete minefield. Brace yourselves, this chapter is going to take me longer to unpick than usual.

Like any other area in the shop, the old adage 'you get what you pay for' holds true for vitamins too. The bargain-priced ultra-cheap tablets will typically contain just enough of each vitamin to meet basic recommendations to prevent severe deficiencies, but there won't be enough supplement power in there to support your body to reach optimal health, especially if levels are already running low.

There has been much scientific investigation into how much or how little of any supplement we really absorb, and often, the better-quality supplements (which inevitably cost more) use expensive formulations your body can absorb and use. Cheaper tablets are so compressed and coated that they might not fully disintegrate and prevent absorption. It has been estimated that tablet absorption can be as low as 30-40% of the advised nutrient content.

I've done ALL the research so you don't have to, and hopefully, once you've read this chapter, you'll be able to scan the vitamin shelves with a bit of an expert eye and pick up the healthiest possible option you can afford.

THE GOOD
Individually prescribed blends of highest possible quality ingredients formulated for maximum absorption.

THE BAD
Cheap, compressed tablets packed with 'fillers', gummies laden with sugar or artificial sweeteners, detox teas and 'fat burners'.

> **THE HEALTHY**
> Clean formulations, max strength doses, minimal
> fillers, and no added sugar. Targeted supplements
> based on individual needs: immunity in winter,
> magnesium for stress/sleep, collagen after the
> age of 30, creatine for muscles and brain.

Sweets in disguise

Vitamin gummies are one of my biggest bugbears, particularly as most of them are heavily marketed at children. Yes, they're fun, tasty and easy to take, but take a look at the label. For many gummies, the first ingredient on the list is sugar or glucose syrup. Many gummy vitamins contain 2-4g of sugar per serving, which can be more than Haribo! Even 'sugar-free' gummies use artificial sweeteners, sugar alcohols or high-sugar fruit juice concentrates to sweeten them. Shameless plug alert: this is why I launched the world's first kids' vitamin gummies made with no added sugar and no sweeteners, using beetroot fibre instead.

Do we really need vitamin supplements anyway?

There's a large body of experts who maintain we don't need supplements because we should be able to get all the nutrients we need from a balanced diet. That might be true – but how many of us eat a perfectly healthy balanced diet? And is the food we eat bursting with nutrition?

You probably won't be getting enough of the right nutrients if you eat highly processed foods which critically are low in nutrition. You'll also struggle to get the nutrients you need if you eat food grown in over-farmed soil that is stripped of its natural nutrients from decades of monocrop farming. And if your stress levels are high (and whose aren't?) your body's nutrient requirements can escalate to levels higher than might be satisfied through food.

Together, these factors can create a perfect storm that leaves our bodies short on essential nutrients. Studies show nine in ten people in the UK aren't getting enough nutrition for optimal bodily health. I was one of those people – even though I ate a supremely healthy diet (you can read more about my story in the intro to this book). This is why I am passionate about fixing nutrition through supplements.

It's ironic – food is everywhere, yet many of us are undernourished. Highly processed and ultra-processed foods dominate our diet. They aren't just bad for us because of all the sugar and additives they contain, but they are critically low in vitamins and minerals too. On top of that, an estimated 31% of our energy intake in the UK comes from cereals and grains, but if you're eating refined white grains, they are relatively devoid of nutrients compared to fruits, vegetables, meat and dairy, and your health is going to be compromised.

Meanwhile, modern agricultural practices have unintentionally lowered the nutrient content of even the healthy foods we do eat. Intensive farming and soil depletion mean that fruits and vegetables today often contain fewer minerals than those grown decades ago. A report comparing UK food composition between 1940 and 2002 found significant declines in mineral content – in some cases up to 70% less vital minerals in our vegetables and fruits.[58] This dilution effect occurs because crops are bred for high yield and they are grown in mineral-exhausted soil; as yield goes up, the concentration of nutrients goes down. In short, the carrot or broccoli on your plate may not be as nutrient-dense as it was in your grandmother's time.

The way we live and handle food further saps nutrients. Back in the day, we would eat food harvested relatively locally, and in season. But now you can easily find yourself eating fruit that has been picked unripe (before those important nutrients have a had a chance to develop) and shipped halfway across the world. Long supply chains and protracted storage can degrade vitamins. Processing and refining often remove nutrient-rich parts of foods too.

We've also got to factor in our modern western lifestyles: chronic stress, lack of sleep, and stimulants like caffeine or alcohol can actually deplete certain nutrients in the body. When you're stressed, your body churns through more magnesium, vitamin C, and B-vitamins to produce stress hormones and keep nerves and muscles functioning.[59]

In other words, modern life not only provides us with LESS nutrition, but it also makes our bodies need MORE nutrition.

Considering these factors, it's not surprising that many adults have measurable nutrient shortfalls. Let's break down the common issues.

A nation of nutrient deficiency

When you look at government or NHS reports, the picture of nutrient deficiency in the UK often looks reassuringly low – usually around 10-20% of people are classed as deficient. But those figures are based on the narrow medical definition of deficiency, where blood levels drop low enough to cause obvious disease. The bigger story is that many more people fall short of what's needed for optimal health, not just to avoid disease. For example, the US-based Linus Pauling Institute's Micronutrient Information Center highlights that, while the RDA is designed as the minimum to prevent deficiency, most people would benefit from aiming for the Optimal Daily Allowance (ODA) – a higher intake that supports long-term wellbeing.[60] By that standard, the majority of UK adults don't consume enough magnesium, vitamin D, iodine, or selenium, and many women are low in folate and iron – even though they're not officially deficient. Put simply: official numbers may look small, but the gap between what we eat and what's ideal is much larger.

The bottom line? It's increasingly hard to get everything you need from diet alone, even if you try to eat well. Our ancestors didn't have to worry about vitamin D drops or magnesium tablets – but they also didn't sit at desks all day, gulp coffee, and eat chips made from potatoes grown in depleted soil. This is where supplements come in. They cannot replace a healthy diet, but they can be a practical tool to bridge the gap between what our bodies need and what modern diets provide.

What supplements do you need?

I always get asked what supplements I take, so I wanted to provide a quick overview of the type of supplements that I think are most relevant for most people and why. This isn't an exhaustive list, and everyone is different: you may have specific needs or deficiencies that you need to focus on. But importantly, each of these is backed by scientific research and reflects documented nutritional issues in the UK population – no overhyped fads make the list!

SWAPS

Cheap multivitamin tablet → High-quality multi with active forms
Better absorption, better outcomes. This is where you have to read the label and look for methylated forms of vitamins.

Gummies → Sugar-free fibre-based gummies
No hidden sugar habit.

Basic fish oil capsules → High-quality omega-3 with no light exposure
Higher EPA (eicosapentaenoic acid) and DHA (docosahexaenoic acid) absorption.

Energy drinks → Creatine + electrolytes
Sustainable strength and hydration without sugar/caffeine crash.

Magnesium oxide (low absorption) → Magnesium citrate or glycinate
Gentler on gut, more bioavailable.

Your nutritional safety net

If you could only take one supplement as 'insurance' for your nutrition, a good multivitamin is the top contender. Multivitamins act as a catch-all because they cover the bases on the essential vitamins and minerals that you might not get every single day. This is especially helpful for people with a poor diet, high UPF consumption or those who eat a lot of takeaways. It's also a great option for certain life stages such as childhood, when consistent good nutrition is critical for development but often hard to achieve. Health authorities recognise the value of broad supplementation in kids: the NHS recommends all children from six months to five years old take daily vitamin A, C, and D supplements.[61]

What can a multivitamin do for you? In practice, people often report having more energy or getting sick less often once they start taking a quality multivitamin, especially if they previously had borderline deficiencies. However, it is important to set realistic expectations: a multi isn't a magic energy pill, but it can subtly improve how you feel by fixing the small nutrient leaks that might be dragging you down.

When choosing a multivitamin, quality counts. Look for a multivitamin that provides high doses at least the full daily value (if not more) of most nutrients. If you see a label, like on some brands, with ten vitamins but with only two at or above 100% nutrient reference value (NRV), then you know it's not going to help. The more nutrients at or above 100% the better. Also look out for active forms of the different nutrients (e.g. folate instead of folic acid, methylcobalamin instead of cyanocobalamin for B12) as these will be better absorbed in the body, but you may have to get your magnifying glass to read the label in detail to spot these.

It is worth considering a multi which is targeted at your specific needs – such as age range and gender. That's because women of childbearing age should have folate to reduce the chance of neural tube defects in case of pregnancy and might want iron in their multi if they have heavy periods, but men often don't need extra iron. Older adults might need more vitamin D and B12. Many brands tailor formulations to these groups.

A multi is your nutritional seat belt – your diet SHOULD cover everything, but the multi is there for backup just in case. Just remember you'll absorb and utilise those extra nutrients best if you take them in conjunction with a healthy balanced diet.

The sunshine vitamin

Vitamin D deserves a special call-out because it's hard to get from food, and the UK's geography and lifestyle put many people at risk of deficiency. Vitamin D is actually a hormone precursor that our skin makes when exposed to UVB sunlight. Up to 90% of our vitamin D intake can come from sun exposure – but in the UK, sun of the right strength is only available for a few summer months. From autumn through to spring, the sun is too weak in this country to trigger vitamin D synthesis, and even in summer we may not get enough sun if we spend all day working or studying indoors.

As a result, vitamin D deficiency is extremely common in the UK. One study highlighted that roughly one-fifth of the UK population is deficient in D, and about 60% have insufficient levels (not full deficiency, but below optimal). Public health officials have taken note and UK guidelines now recommend everyone consider taking a vitamin D supplement, especially in the winter months. The usual suggestion is 10 micrograms (400IU) daily for adults, though many experts argue this is a bare minimum and that 25-50 micrograms (1,000-2,000IU) daily might be more ideal for adults to reach optimal blood levels.

Why does vitamin D matter so much? For decades we only talked about D in the context of bones – it's crucial for calcium absorption, so without enough D, children could get rickets (soft, deformed bones) and adults can be vulnerable to osteoporosis. But now we know vitamin D receptors exist all over the body, including in the immune system, brain, and other tissues. Vitamin D plays a role in immune support, helping the body fend off infections. In skin health, adequate vitamin D helps maintain the skin barrier and can ward off inflammatory issues. And there's ongoing research into vitamin D's role in mood.

For UK adults, supplementing vitamin D is almost a no-brainer, especially through the winter. Vitamin D3 (cholecalciferol) is the preferred form (it's the same form that your body makes from sunlight), typically sourced from lanolin in sheep's wool, though vegan D3 from lichen (a plant moss) is available. Taking it with a meal that has some fat can help absorption. Check the vitamin

D levels in your multi. If they're not adequate, you may need to take a specific pill.

Skin, hair and nails

Collagen has become a buzzword in wellness circles, but in my opinion (which is, of course, backed up by science) it's not just hype. Collagen is literally the most abundant protein in our bodies, acting like a structural glue in our skin, joints, and connective tissues. Our bodies produce collagen naturally, but here's the truth: after the age of 30, our collagen production starts to slow down, and existing collagen fibres begin to break down faster. In fact, it's estimated we lose roughly 1% of our collagen per year from early adulthood. Women experience a particularly sharp drop in collagen synthesis in the first few years of menopause (losing up to 30% of skin collagen in about five years post-menopause). This decline in collagen is a major reason we see skin ageing and why joints might get stiffer as we get older.

Collagen supplements typically come in the form of powders or capsules containing hydrolysed collagen peptides (broken-down collagen proteins, often sourced from bovine or marine collagen). The idea is that these supplements can give your body the building blocks to shore up and stimulate collagen production in skin, cartilage, etc. Does it work? Research is still ongoing, but a number of randomised controlled trials[62] have shown promising results for skin health: oral collagen supplements have been found to improve skin hydration, elasticity, and even reduce wrinkle depth according to systematic reviews. There are different types of collagens you will find. Marine collagen usually provides mainly type I (great for skin, hair and nails), bovine collagen contains both type I and III (skin, muscles, and blood vessels), and chicken collagen is often rich in type II (best known for supporting joints and cartilage).

For joint health, Knaub et al[63] found type II collagen shows benefits in reducing joint pain and improving joint function. It makes sense: collagen is a major component of cartilage, which provides the cushioning for our joints. There's also emerging interest in collagen for bone health since bones are about one-third collagen by mass – it's what gives them flexibility.

In practical terms, collagen supplements might be worth considering if:

- You're over 30 and starting to notice skin ageing or joint aches, and you want to be proactive.
- You're very physically active (e.g. a runner or weightlifter) putting stress on joints and connective tissues.

Collagen powder is easy to incorporate – it usually dissolves into coffee, smoothies, or oatmeal with minimal taste. A typical dose is around 5-10g daily.

One thing to manage expectations: don't expect overnight miracles. Collagen supplements tend to show results after 1-3 months of consistent use. And individuals with very balanced diets rich in protein might not see as dramatic an effect as someone who had a poor diet to begin with. But given that collagen production undeniably declines with age and that our dietary intake of collagen (which we once might have got from bone broth, slow-cooked meats with connective tissue, or fish skin) is usually low in modern diets, supplementing can be a convenient way to ensure you have those specific peptides handy for your body to use.

Great sleep and muscle relaxation

Magnesium doesn't always get the attention it deserves, but it's a quiet hero mineral that's involved in hundreds of enzymatic reactions in the body (over 300, by most counts). From energy production to muscle relaxation, nerve signalling, blood pressure regulation, and even the synthesis of our DNA – magnesium is busy behind the scenes in almost every system of the body. Perhaps most relevant to the average person, magnesium is known as nature's relaxant: it helps calm the nervous system, relax muscle, and can even play a role in mood regulation.

When you're under chronic stress (whether that's physical or emotional), your body powers through magnesium reserves at a higher rate because magnesium is used to quell the adrenaline response and mitigate the effects of stress hormones. You can easily get caught in a vicious cycle whereby stress depletes magnesium, but low magnesium makes you more susceptible to the negative effects of stress (such as anxiety, poor sleep, muscle tension) as demonstrated by Pickering et al.[64] No wonder magnesium is often recommended for people who feel 'tired but wired,' have trouble sleeping, or suffer muscle cramps and headaches – all of which are possible signs of a magnesium shortfall.

Problems can arise because magnesium is one of the key minerals that many of us don't get enough of from food. You'll get plenty of magnesium in your diet if you eat whole grains, leafy greens, nuts, seeds, and legumes – but far too few people do. Plus, modern farming's soil depletion has hit magnesium content hard, since it's not one of the three nutrients added in common fertilizers. According to data from the US National Health and Nutrition Examination Survey (NHANES), approximately 61% of adults in the United States consume less magnesium than the RDA.[65]

When choosing a magnesium supplement, the form does matter. Better forms include magnesium citrate and magnesium glycinate, as these are more bioavailable and gentler on the gut.

The bottom line is magnesium is a foundational mineral to consider supplementing, given how prevalent low intakes are. If you're part of the 61% of people who might be running low, getting your magnesium in order could pay dividends in terms of better sleep, steadier mood, and smoother functioning all around. Given the elemental size of magnesium, this is also something that should be taken in addition to your multi as you'll never find a multi with 300mg of magnesium, which is an optimal level.

Supercharge your fluid intake

Drinking enough fluid and taking on the right balance of electrolytes is crucial for day-to-day wellbeing, especially for those with active lifestyles. Electrolytes (such as sodium, potassium, magnesium, calcium, chloride) are specific minerals that carry an electric charge in our body fluids. They help maintain fluid balance, enable proper nerve conduction (that's how your brain talks to your muscles), and allow muscles (including your heart) to contract and relax normally. If you've ever been dehydrated or sweated heavily, you might have felt dizzy, headachey, experienced muscle cramps, or just felt mentally foggy – those are signs of electrolyte imbalance.

Many of us walk around mildly dehydrated without realising it. We might drink plenty of tea or coffee, but those can act as diuretics, meaning we excrete more liquid than we take on. Far too many of us simply don't drink enough plain water throughout the day. A busy office worker might forget to hydrate until they feel thirsty (by which time they're already slightly dehydrated). And active individuals – say you go to the gym, or for a run, or even a sweaty yoga class – lose not just water but also sodium and other electrolytes through sweat. Rehydrating with plain water alone after intense exercise or prolonged sweating can dilute your remaining electrolytes and sometimes isn't enough to fully restore optimal levels.

Even mild dehydration has measurable effects on your body and brain. A study by Baker et al[66] shows that being just 1-2% dehydrated led to worsened mood, fatigue, and headaches. Other studies[67] have noted that around 2%

dehydration caused difficulty in tasks requiring concentration and increased anxiety/tension. In athletes, as little as 1.5% dehydration was shown to reduce strength and power output significantly, and 2%+ dehydration clearly hinders endurance performance. The trick is this is so little that most of us wouldn't even realise we haven't hydrated properly.

Water and electrolytes are like the oil in your car – easy to overlook, but things start misfiring without them.

For most people, aiming to drink a good 1.5 to 2 litres of fluid a day (more if it's hot or if you exercise) is a solid goal. But it could be worth adding electrolytes in to aid optimal bodily function.

Many commercial sports drinks are basically sugar water with a dash of salt, which is not ideal. Look for formulations with no added sugar or only minimal sugar, and which provide a balanced mix of the key electrolytes – sodium is number one for rehydration, but potassium, magnesium, chloride and calcium are important too. Rehydrating with electrolytes can refresh your body and clear the 'fog' in your mind in a way plain water sometimes doesn't. It's a simple supplement tweak you can make that will deliver noticeable results.

Power trip

If there's one sports supplement that has transcended gym bros and become universally respected, it's creatine. Creatine monohydrate (the most common form) is a favourite for weightlifters and athletes because of its well-documented ability to boost muscle power and growth. Indeed, creatine is one of the most studied supplements in the world, with research consistently showing that supplementing with creatine (typically 3-5g daily) can lead to significant improvements in muscle strength, power output, and lean muscle mass when you're regularly resistance training. Essentially, creatine helps your muscles recycle their energy currency (ATP) faster during high-intensity efforts, allowing you to squeeze out that extra rep or sprint a bit faster, which over time translates to better gains.

Now, here's the part you might not know: creatine isn't just good for muscles, it also benefits the brain. Research has emerged showing the cognitive benefits of creatine supplementation. For instance, a systematic review of trials found that creatine intake may improve short-term memory and intelligence/reasoning tasks, particularly in people who are sleep-deprived or stressed. Some studies showed vegetarians (who often have lower baseline creatine since meat is a primary source) registered improved memory after taking creatine, and older adults might see cognitive perks too.

In general, if you engage in any kind of regular exercise – be it weight training, HIIT classes, sports, or even heavy gardening on weekends – creatine can help you perform better and recover better. If you're not very active, creatine may not be as immediately necessary, but some recent research suggests it could still help with muscle preservation and cognitive function in older people, even if they're not hitting the gym, by supporting overall cellular energy.

Five grams a day is the standard dose. Some do a

'loading phase' of around 20g/day for a week to saturate muscle stores faster, but it's not strictly needed; you'll reach saturation in about 3-4 weeks just taking 5g daily. Creatine dissolves in water or can be mixed into your post-workout shake. Make sure to stay well-hydrated when on creatine, as your muscles will be drawing in a bit more water – which is part of how it works. It's a trusted supplement with proven benefits for strength and muscle health, and exciting potential benefits for brain health.

Supplements are not magic bullets, but they can effectively counteract the less-than-ideal aspects of our diet and lifestyle today. A sugar-laden chewable vitamin might not be much better than candy, but a thoughtfully chosen supplement could fill critical gaps and optimise your health. You stand to benefit most from focusing on the fundamentals: covering common deficiencies (like D and magnesium), supporting overall diet quality (multivitamin), addressing age-related changes (collagen), keeping hydrated (electrolytes), and fuelling muscle and brain function (creatine).

As always, one should consider individual needs and possibly consult with a healthcare provider, especially if you have any health conditions or take medications. But for most healthy adults, the supplements discussed are low-risk and high-reward when used appropriately.

Below is a quick guide so you can see what is right for you:

Supplement	Who it's for?	Why take it?	UK deficiency risk	How to use it
Multivitamin	Anyone with a less-than-ideal diet, kids, picky eaters, dieters.	Covers nutrient gaps. Supports energy and all-round health.	Common shortfalls in D, B12, iron, magnesium, zinc.	Take daily with food. Choose high-quality, natural forms. Kids under five need vitamins A, C, D as per NHS guidelines.
Vitamin D (D3)	Everyone in UK (especially Sept–Mar), office workers, older adults, those with darker skin.	Supports bone health, energy and winter immunity.	~20% deficient, 60% insufficient.	Take 10–50 µg daily. D3 with food. Be consistent daily.
Collagen	Over-30s, those noticing skin ageing, joint strain, or injury recovery.	Supports skin elasticity, joint health, and nail/hair strength.	Production drops ~1% yearly from adulthood.	5-10g / day in a drink. Combine with vitamin C. Give it 8-12 weeks to work.
Magnesium	Athletes, headache, PMS sufferers, plus anyone who is stressed, anxious, sleeping poorly.	Calms nerves, improves sleep, aids recovery, lowers blood pressure.	Likely 61%+ suboptimal intake.	300mg/day, preferably at night. Use glycinate/citrate forms. Epsom baths also helpful.
Electrolytes	Exercisers, heavy sweaters, sauna users, tired/foggy, or don't drink enough water.	Rehydrates, prevents cramps, supports energy and focus	Mild dehydration very common.	Use in/after exercise or during 3pm slump. Drink steadily. Adjust to sweat level.

Supplement	Who it's for?	Why take it?	UK deficiency risk	How to use it
Creatine	Gym-goers, vegetarians, working adults, students under stress.	Boosts strength, muscle growth, mental clarity, reduces fatigue.	No clinical deficiency, low intake in non-meat eaters/ older adults	5g daily. Stay hydrated.

(Sources: NHS guidelines, UK nutrition surveys, and referenced scientific studies throughout this chapter, among others.)

Packing in the protein

When we're trying to eat healthily, we've all probably grabbed a protein bar or shake as a quick fix. I remember back in the day, whenever I threw myself into a new training plan at the gym or was about to kick-start a new three-month programme, I'd always buy a box of protein bars as motivation and a way to help me bulk up. I was convinced I needed them. It is true that, when you train, you need to consume more protein, but I now know that by buying protein bars, I was missing the point.

I thought the added protein was the key to muscle building, but the truth is it's actually far more important to be consistent with your training and food intake than it is to add some magic protein supplement.

Today, walk into any UK supermarket or shop and you'll see Grenade bars, Huel shakes, Fulfil bars and more

– all promising to deliver a much-needed protein hike. Yes, they are convenient, and they certainly taste great, but these ultra-processed protein snacks simply don't stack up against old-school protein sources such as eggs, cheese, or nuts.

And it's not just bars and shakes. 'High-protein' has become a marketing buzzword stamped onto all sorts of everyday foods, from breads and cereals to pastas and even crisps. But here's the catch: when you check the labels, the actual protein increase compared to the standard version is often only 30% more, while the price tag might be as high as 50% more. To make matters worse, boosting the protein usually means adding protein isolates or concentrates, which is another layer of processing that doesn't necessarily improve the overall nutritional quality.

In this chapter, I'll set popular protein products against non-ultra-processed protein sources and compare cost, protein content, satiety, and overall nutritional quality. The results might surprise you.

THE GOOD
Real food: meat, fish, dairy products and legumes.

THE BAD
Ultra-processed protein products packed with artificial sweeteners, gums, and oils.

THE HEATHLY
Natural protein supplements such as Form Nutrition, the Organic Protein Company, and WillPowders with no artificial sweeteners or gums.

Pricey protein

Let's start with the protein punch per pound. Those shiny packaged snacks tend to be pricey for the protein they deliver. Consider a few examples:

- **Grenade Carb Killa Bar (60g)** – roughly 12p per gram of protein.
- **Fulfil Protein Bar (40g)** – around 13p per protein gram.
- **Huel Ready-to-Drink (500ml)** – roughly 17.5p per gram of protein.
- Now compare those to real food sources readily found in your fridge or local Tesco:
- **Eggs (around 58g each)** – about 5p per gram of protein (eggs come packed with vitamins and minerals to boot).
- **Cheddar cheese** – roughly 3.2p per protein gram (along with calcium and other nutrients).
- **Peanuts** (or other nuts) – about 3p per gram of protein – plus healthy fats, fibre, and micronutrients.

It's simple maths, but these protein bars and ready-made shakes cost easily four or five times more per gram of protein than the natural protein you get from an egg or a handful of nuts. When you hand over your cash, you're largely paying for marketing, convenience, and pretty packaging.

If you're on a budget, it's clear that real foods give you much more protein for your money. For the price of one protein bar, you could buy a dozen eggs or nearly half a kilo of peanuts. Real foods fill you up for longer, too. The protein and fat in real foods such as eggs, cheese, and nuts work together to contribute to lasting satiety. These foods require more chewing, which slows your digestion down and gives your body time to register fullness. By contrast, it's easy to demolish a sweet chocolate-flavoured protein bar in seconds, and you may find yourself feeling hungry again soon afterwards.

Swift swaps when you're on the move:

SWAPS

Protein bar → Hard-boiled eggs
Every store with a meal deal has them. They are cheaper and more protein-rich without the additives.

Protein shake → Slices of cheese
Available in most stores with a fridge, double the protein content, none of the artificial sweeteners and a similar price.

Protein snack → Peanuts
Available everywhere and incredibly affordable and versatile. If you can get baked not fried ones you are onto a protein winner without the junk.

Protein powders

Walk into any health aisle and you'll see giant tubs of protein powder stacked like trophies. Whey, soy, pea, hemp – all promising leaner muscles and faster recovery. And yes, powders do offer a quick, convenient way to boost your protein intake, especially if you struggle to hit your daily needs through food alone like I often do. About 1.6-2g of protein per kg of bodyweight is ideal for muscle growth. My weight tends to hover at around 80kg so I'm looking for 160g of protein from my food per day. A scoop of protein powder stirred into milk can easily add 20-25g protein to that daily total, which is great and convenient, but there are a ton of additives to watch out for.

Many mainstream protein powder blends are packed with artificial sweeteners, gums, flavourings, and emulsifiers to make them creamier and more addictive. The label might make them look delicious but the ingredients list often reads like a chemistry experiment.

THE GOOD
Use powders sparingly and occasionally to top up protein. Instead, focus on wholefood sources like eggs, dairy, nuts, fish as your optimal daily foundation.

THE BAD
Flavoured protein powder blends with long lists of chemical ingredients including gums and sweeteners.

THE HEALTHY
Pure whey or plant powders with short ingredients lists, no artificial sweeteners or gums.

What's really inside?

One protein bar I found delivers 21g of protein, mostly from milk, which isn't in itself bad, but the ingredients list also includes the artificial sweeteners maltitol and sucralose, alongside 21 other compounds including palm oil, rapeseed oil, polydextrose, emulsifier, wheat starch and flavouring. This particular bar is marketed as healthy – 'high-protein, low-sugar' – because it has only 1g of sugar. But the sweet taste comes from artificial additives, which might have fewer calories but which can cause bloating or a laxative effect.

There's a growing clarity in nutrition science that it's not just macros (the proteins, carbohydrates, fats) that matter to our health, but the food matrix and the way nutrients are bundled together.

With real foods, what you see is what you get. As well as protein, an egg contains natural nutrients such as choline, vitamin D, and selenium that come packaged by nature, without additives. Cheese is basically fermented milk with salt – a good source of calcium and protein, with no ingredients list full of chemicals. Nuts come with fibre, magnesium, and healthy fats intact.

Protein bars and shakes do have their place – they're convenient and portable. If you're in a rush or need a quick protein hit immediately after a workout, grabbing something in a package or a bottle might be better than nothing. But it's worth keeping perspective: you'll be paying a hefty premium for that convenience, and you're consuming a product that is, by definition, engineered and ultra-processed.

Most people, most of the time, are better off getting their protein from real foods. Use those convenient protein products strategically (when travelling or in a pinch), but remember that an egg, a piece of cheese, or a handful of nuts can often do the same job better – with more nutrients, more satiety, and far less processing.

CLEANING SWAPS

THE DAILY CLEAN

As you reach for your bottles of bleach, surface spray, limescale remover or washing-up liquid and throw them into your shopping trolley, the chances are you're thinking about keeping your house clean and not worrying about your health.

I used to buy whatever was on deal and not pay too much attention to this stuff, until I started to learn more about the chemicals they contain. It's pretty scary when you learn where these nasties end up, how our body is exposed to them, and the health impacts this can have.

Flip over a typical bottle of washing-up liquid or laundry detergent and you are likely to find a warning: 'Harmful to aquatic life with long-lasting effects'. This exact label appears on everything from Fairy washing-up liquid to Persil laundry capsules and plenty of other common brands in between. These warnings aren't just for show; they state overtly the real environmental risks of pouring harsh and toxic chemicals down the drain. Yet that's exactly what we do with them. Day in and day out.

I don't think enough of us realise that the chemicals that scrub our plates and clothes clean can wreak havoc once we flush them away, as well as causing issues for our own skin.

So come with me. Let's uncover the science behind their impacts and explore safer, greener alternatives.

THE GOOD
Plant-based products made with biodegradable surfactants to help reduce chemicals from polluting our environment.

THE BAD
Mainstream dishwashing liquids, pods, and laundry detergents which contain petroleum surfactants, PVA film, artificial dyes, fragrances, and known irritants such as methylisothiazolinone.

THE HEALTHY
Plastic-free dishwasher tablets, old-fashioned powder detergents in cardboard boxes, wool dryer balls instead of softeners, and fragrance-free plant-based products.

Hands that do dishes

Washing-up liquid is a kitchen staple, but its ingredients can be harsher than you'd expect. Mainstream UK brands rely on surfactants derived from fossil fuels. These are the chemicals that cut grease and produce lots of foam. The trouble is that these same surfactants don't simply vanish after we've cleaned the dishes. When you pull the plug, the waste water carries those compounds out of your home to treatment works, but traces eventually end up in rivers and oceans. This is especially true during bad storms, when parts of the UK's sewer system use overflows that bypass the usual treatment methods and flow straight into our rivers and seas. Studies have shown that common surfactants can linger in waterways, where they are toxic to marine life.[68] Experts writing in the

Journal of Applied Microbiology even went as far as to say: 'Surfactants are capable of penetrating the cell membrane and thus cause toxicity to living organisms. Accumulation of these compounds has been known to cause significant gill damage and loss of sight in fish.'

It's not just fish that can feel the effects. The same detergents that are tough on grime can also be tough on your skin. Fairy Liquid contains methylisothiazolinone, which was banned in the EU in 2017 for 'leave-on cosmetic products' like lotions and creams, due to concerns that it could irritate the skin, yet your daily dish soap is allowed to contain it because the expectation is that you rinse your hands after washing up. But it may still cause skin irritation. Even consumer giants like L'Oreal have said, 'We have decided to go beyond the regulation and to completely phase out methylisothiazolinone in our products, including rinse-off products.'[69] If you've ever finished a sink full of dishes only to find your hands dry, red or itchy, the detergent could be to blame.

The good news is that cleaning up your dish-washing routine is relatively easy. A wave of plant-based, eco-friendly washing-up liquids are available for not too dissimilar prices, offering effective cleaning without the nasties. Brands like Ecover, Bio-D, Method, and Greenscents formulate their dish soaps with biodegradable plant-based ingredients and without petroleum surfactants. Many of these alternatives are also free of added dyes and fragrances, making them gentler on sensitive skin. For example, Ecover's Zero washing-up liquid is fragrance-free and dermatologically tested, so it's tough on grease yet gentle on your skin and the waterways.

SWAPS

Fairy Liquid → Plant-based washing-up liquid
Same grease-cutting power, biodegradable ingredients, no harsh skin irritants.

The dish on dishwasher tablets

If you're not bothered too much about washing-up liquid because you've got a dishwasher to do the dirty work, there are still issues to be addressed. Your hands might be safe from damage, but dishwasher detergents can still pose a hidden environmental cost. If you're using popular dishwasher tablets or pods, you've probably tried those little capsules wrapped in a shiny, dissolvable film. They're extra-convenient because they don't have to be unwrapped. They are encased in a synthetic polymer that dissolves in the wash. It's tempting to think these single-dose pods are magically waste-free. After all, the plastic film seems to 'disappear' in water, but emerging research shows that's not the full story. When PVA film dissolves, it doesn't simply turn into water and air; it forms a micro-scopic plastic solution that flows out with the wastewater. The conditions in a typical wastewater treatment facility are not ideal for breaking down PVA completely. In fact, a recent analysis found that about 75% of the PVA from detergent pods survives the treatment process and passes into the environment.[70] Essentially, tons of microplastic bits from our dishwashers are making their way into rivers and oceans. Another study, this one in the *International Journal of Environmental Research and Public Health* quoted 'massive production numbers make it a cause for concern as a pollutant in the natural environment,' so, this might be adding up to tons of PVA pollution released annually given their frequent use in most households.[71]

Once in the environment, these dissolved plastics join other microplastics in entering the food chain. It's a similar issue to the plastic microbeads that were once common in cosmetics and were banned due to their environmental impact.

The good news is, it's super-easy to reduce your impact on the environment without giving up the convenience. Simply ditch the dissolvable plastic pods. There are plenty of options that use no PVA film. Notably, in 2025 Ecover launched an industry-first plastic-free dishwasher tablet, with a coating that contains no PVA at all. These tablets come packed in cardboard and they deliver the same cleaning power without the microplastics. By opting for these, you can prevent that hidden plastic from ever entering the water system.

While you're hunting through the more environmentally friendly options in this aisle of the supermarket, look for plant-based dishwasher detergents. Companies like Ecover offer dishwasher powder or tablets that use biodegradable, plant-derived enzymes and surfactants to break down food residue in your machine.

SWAPS

**Dishwasher pods wrapped in dissolvable plastic →
Plastic-free dishwasher tablets**
Stop thousands of tonnes of microplastics from
entering waterways each year.

**Plastic-free dishwasher tablets → Plant-based plastic-
free dishwasher tablets/powder**

Clean clothes, clean planet

Now let's focus on the washing machine, and I bet you now know what I'm going to say. Yes, laundry products ALSO have a way of sneaking chemical residues into both our environment and our daily lives. The problem is, conventional laundry detergents often contain a cocktail of potent cleaning agents: surfactants, stain removers, optical brighteners, artificial fragrances, dyes, and more. While these ingredients can make your clothes look and smell impeccably clean, they don't always play nice with the world outside your washing machine (or with people who have sensitive skin).

One major concern is (once more) the plastic film on laundry pods which contain the same PVA that leaches into the waterways, contributing to the microplastics load which disrupts the delicate environmental balance.

An additional laundry pollutant to consider is the millions of microscopic microfibres that shed from synthetic fabrics as they tumble around in your washing machine. These tiny fibres wash out of our clothes and end up in waterways too. Together, these two factors make laundry day a surprisingly big microplastics contributor.

Of course, all the chemicals used in laundry products are regulated and deemed safe to use, but many are sufficiently caustic to cause skin problems for people with sensitive skins. Research shows that detergents can leave chemical residues in fabrics even after they've been properly rinsed. These residues may include irritants such as synthetic fragrance compounds and other additives. One major study found '162 fragrances that have been reported to cause contact allergy/allergic contact dermatitis'.[72] Prolonged exposure to such chemicals against the skin can trigger contact dermatitis or exacerbate conditions such as eczema. No wonder many people with sensitive skin or parents of small children choose 'non-bio' and fragrance-free laundry products as a protective measure.

From an environmental perspective, whatever doesn't stay in your clothes goes down the drain. Laundry wastewater carries detergent chemicals out to sewage treatment works, and though the majority are removed, some ingredients persist. As with dish products, any phosphates (if present) can contribute to issues in our rivers like uncontrolled algae growth. The surfactants and other chemicals, if not biodegradable, can accumulate and harm aquatic life.

Thankfully again, there are good alternatives. Plant-based laundry detergents offer a compelling solution to conventional soaps that work just as well. When shopping for greener laundry options, look for labels like fragrance-free, plant-based, biodegradable, or certifications from organisations like Allergy UK or EcoCert. This is starting to sound like an Ecover advert now, but they are one of the most widely available good options. Their Zero range includes a non-bio laundry liquid that has no added fragrance or colours and is endorsed by Allergy UK for sensitive skin. UK brands such as Bio-D, Faith in Nature, and even some supermarket eco lines offer similar products. These detergents prove that you can get rid of stubborn stains and odours without the need for harsh chemicals. You may also consider old-fashioned powder detergents in cardboard boxes – powders often have fewer additives than liquids and the packaging is plastic-free.

SWAPS

Liquid laundry pods → Old-fashioned laundry powder
Fewer additives, less plastic, cardboard packaging.

Fabric softeners → Wool dryer balls
To soften clothes and reduce static, optionally with a couple of drops of natural essential oil for light scent.

Stain removers (which contain chlorine, bleach or chemical brighteners) → Sodium bicarbonate or baking soda
Can be used to whiten and remove stains.

Making the switch to greener cleaning products for your home is a win for you and the environment. By replacing a few staple products, you can significantly reduce the chemical and plastic footprint of your daily chores. So, let's clean up our cleaning habits.

COOKWARE
SWAPS

COOKING EQUIPMENT

Most of us don't think about cooking equipment while we're rushing around the supermarket doing our weekly shop, but in the interest of your health, it might be time to add a few new hardware items to your shopping list.

For instance, if your trusty frying pan is beginning to look a bit scratched, buying a replacement might be the kitchen intervention your health needs. Non-stick cookware, often coated with Teflon, has been a hero for hassle-free cooking for many years, but it comes with a dark secret. Older non-stick pans were made with a chemical called PFOA, which is part of a family of 'forever chemicals' called PFAS that have been banned in the UK since 2005. Research had linked peeling non-stick coatings and the microplastic bits they shed with health issues such as hormonal disruption and even increased cancer risk.

Your non-stick pan may not be quite that old, but there are still concerns to consider. Modern Teflon pans no longer use PFOA, but they use other chemicals which they maintain are safe at normal cooking temperatures. But even these improved coatings have challenges. The danger is wear-and-tear. Cranking the heat too high (above around 260 °C) can overheat the coating, causing it to break down and release toxic fumes. People talk about 'Teflon flu', flu-like symptoms that can be caused by inhaling fumes from an empty pan left on max. It's good to watch out for physical damage too. A single scratch on a Teflon pan could shed over 9,000 microplastic particles into your dinner according to a recent study.[73] 'It gives us a strong warning that we must be careful about selecting and using cooking utensils to avoid food contamination,' says Professor Tang, from the College of Science and Engineering at Flinders University in Australia. So, avoid using metal implements which might scratch your nonstick pan.

The reason PFAS are called 'forever chemicals' is because they don't biodegrade. Instead, they accumulate in our environment and bodies over time, potentially messing with our hormones, fertility, and immune systems. Even the government is waking up to this by appointing the Environmental Audit Committee to launch an inquiry into PFAS in 2025. The committee chair, Toby Perkins MP, said: 'PFAS forever chemicals are prevalent in countless everyday items. News coverage has exposed the level of problems with PFAS, and has shone a light that the UK's regulatory approach is far less active than in many other jurisdictions.' Your old frying pan won't hurt you today, but it's wise to be aware of the long-term problems it might be contributing to.

The good news is you can enjoy the slippery convenience of a non-stick pan without the sketchy chemicals. Ceramic-coated pans, for example, use a silica-based coating (similar to glass or sand) to ensure your fried eggs slide off with ease, no Teflon in sight. Major manufacturers like GreenPan and even Tefal sell ceramic non-stick ranges that are PFOA/PFAS-free but still deliver on slipperiness. Just treat them properly, avoiding metal utensils or abrasive scrubbers, and they'll serve you well.

> **THE GOOD**
> Cast iron, naturally non-stick with seasoning,
> and stainless steel – durable, non-toxic.
>
> **THE BAD**
> Old, scratched non-stick cookware shedding
> microplastics and PFAS.
>
> **THE HEALTHY**
> Modern and ceramic-coated pans which are
> marked as PFAS-free. Use carefully at low heat.
> Convenient but not long-lasting.

I'm a big fan of old-school cast iron. Those pans develop a natural non-stick coating over time with seasoning, and they can outlast you! Seasoning a cast iron pan is the process of creating a natural, non-stick coating by applying a thin layer of oil and heating it until it forms a hard, protective surface that enhances cooking performance. Unlike synthetic coatings such as Teflon, seasoning is chemical-free and that non-stick layer can be built up over time with regular use. You can literally leave a cast iron pan outside in the rain to rust for years, bring it inside, sand off the rust, and then season it again with oil and you'll be good to go.

Stainless steel pans are another kitchen workhorse because they are completely non-toxic, durable, and great for high-heat searing. You might need an extra drizzle of oil to prevent sticking, and make sure you heat the pan before putting food in, but you'll get superb browning and a pan that can go from hob to oven easily. That's why high-end chefs love them.

So, what's the catch on cost? Non-stick pans may be cheap, but if you've got to replace them every few years, the costs can mount. Cast iron and stainless steel, on the other hand, can last a lifetime. If cared for and used often, they can be passed down through family generations.

Ditch the plastic spatula

If your plastic spatulas have become a bit warped on the edges, or the handles on your big plastic spoon scarred from resting on a hot pan, there's every chance they're shedding teeny tiny plastic particles into your food. Recent studies show that plastic utensils can be another area you need to avoid. Dr Amy Lusher of NIVA Norway said, 'Our results were concerning – showing that plastic cookware is likely adding thousands of microplastics into the human diet each year'.[74] Heat makes it worse: stir a boiling curry with a cheap plastic spoon and you may be leaching not only plastic bits but also chemicals within the plastic into that curry. Plastics are made with additives such as plasticisers for flexibility, flame retardants, and dyes. When the plastic is heated or scratched, those extras can migrate out into your dinner.

THE GOOD
Wooden, bamboo, or stainless-steel utensils:
safe and durable.

> **THE BAD**
> Old black plastic utensils which release toxins
> and microplastics when hot.
>
> **THE HEALTHY**
> Newer BPA-free plastics, but only when used
> briefly with low heat.

Flame retardants are added to some black plastic utensils to make them more resistant to catching fire. That might be good for your immediate safety, but not so much in the long-term. Some are also made from recycled electronics plastics that contained flame retardants. Scientists detected these chemicals in 85% of black plastic kitchen utensils tested.[75] The UK has banned many flame retardants due to concerns about their potential harm to human health and the environment. Some were linked to cancer, thyroid and hormone disruption, and developmental issues, so production ceased in 1996. Yet those flame retardants could still find their way into your kitchen cupboard through a recycled black plastic spoon that might have come from an old electronic device.

Other common plasticisers such as BPA (bisphenol A) or phthalates can sneak into your food from plastic kitchen implements, especially if they're exposed to high heat. These act as endocrine disruptors, basically confusing your hormones – which is why BPA is banned from water bottles. The sad fact remains, however, that a 'BPA-free' label could just mean an equally toxic chemical cousin is lurking in there instead.

Fortunately, Mother Nature has our backs. Wooden

and bamboo utensils are fantastic alternatives. A wooden spoon won't leach oestrogen-mimickers into your stew. Wood is gentle on cookware surfaces and is completely biodegradable when it eventually retires. Bamboo is similar: lightweight, durable, and often cheaply available. You can grab a set of bamboo spoons and spatulas cheaply online or at any home goods store. Chopping or stirring with bamboo won't generate microplastics – one study found that meat cut on a bamboo cutting board had zero plastic fragments, while the same job on a plastic board dished up hundreds of microscopic particles.[76] It's clear: natural materials play nicer with our food.

Another stalwart option is stainless steel utensils. Steel tongs, spoons, and spatulas can handle heat beyond anything your stove can throw at them, and they don't introduce any weird chemicals, so they're perfect for use with stainless steel or cast iron cookware. The only caveat: don't use metal on non-stick pans as you'll scratch that coating right off, but if you're reading this, hopefully you've thrown out your non-stick pans by now!

SWAPS

Plastic spatula → Bamboo or wooden spoon
Ditch hormone-disrupting chemicals for
biodegradable simplicity.

Let's talk microplastics and your health – why do we care about a few tiny plastic specks anyway? The problem is these particles are turning up everywhere – in human blood, lungs, even placentas. Early research suggests they might provoke inflammation, carry toxic substances, or mess with our gut microbiomes. It's still a developing science, but I'd rather not be part of that experiment if I can help it. 'All of us need to stop using plastic as much as we can to protect our health, especially single-use plastics,' said Desiree LaBeaud, a physician at Stanford Medicine, in the US, who founded the Plastics and Health Working Group.[77] Upgrading your utensils is low-cost and your body will thank you later.

Beware the tupperware avalanche

In every kitchen there will be one cupboard overflowing with mismatched plastic containers, a.k.a. the Tupperware avalanche. These plastic tubs are super-handy for leftovers, packed lunches, and freezing meals but they can introduce unwanted extras into your food, especially when heated. If you've noticed your old takeaway containers are permanently orange-tinted and carry a whiff of last week's curry, here's why: plastics can absorb colours and oils, and in turn leach chemicals back into your food when re-used, scratched, or heated. That stain isn't just a cosmetic issue – it's a sign the plastic has broken down a bit. And when that happens, chemical compounds can migrate into whatever food you store in there.

THE GOOD
Glass or stainless-steel containers.

THE BAD
Old, damaged plastic containers in the microwave.

THE HEALTHY
BPA-free plastics for cold storage only.

Many manufacturers voluntarily pulled BPA from food containers due to public pressure and 'BPA-free' labels are now plastered on everything from water bottles to lunchboxes. However the chemicals replacing BPA (such as BPS or BPF) may be just as likely to mess with our hormones. All plastics can release small amounts of chemicals when heated. Even Cancer Research UK, while reassuring that normal use of plastic containers isn't a cancer risk, notes that some chemicals can migrate into food during microwaving.[78]

Heat is the catalyst here. Microwaving plastic is convenient – we've all done the 'lid ajar' reheat of yesterday's lasagne – but it's not great for the container or for you. High heat can cause the plastic polymer chains to break down slightly, releasing plasticisers or other additives into the food. One study found that filling a disposable polypropylene cup with near-boiling water (95°C) released 50% more microplastic particles into the water compared to a cup filled with warm (50°C) water.[79] If you've ever pulled a warped lid or a container that's gone soft out of the microwave, that's physical proof that the plastic is degrading and invisible chemicals are likely to have leached into the food.

Time for change. Glass storage containers are a game-changer. Glass is completely non-reactive, meaning it won't absorb smells or stains, and it won't release any chemical compounds into your food. You can safely microwave glass. The only downsides to glass are weight and breakability – they're heavier to carry, and if you drop one, well, you know the story. But treat them well, and they'll last indefinitely.

If you are looking to save on weight for school lunches or your backpack, another alternative is stainless steel food containers. Steel is durable, won't stain or retain odours, and it doesn't leach any nasties. You can't microwave steel, so these are best for storage and transport. But for salads, sandwiches or snacks they're brilliant. They're also light and unbreakable. A high-quality stainless lunchbox might cost you a bit more than plastic, but it's virtually indestructible and can last you a lifetime.

For the uber eco-friendly folks, there are also reusable silicone zip bags that can replace disposable plastic bags for snacks and fridge/freezer storage. These are quite durable and dishwasher safe. Just ensure you are buying 100% food-grade silicone. Beeswax wraps are a good swap for clingfilm. These malleable cloths coated in beeswax can be pressed over bowls or around sandwiches. They don't work for liquids or long-term storage, but they're great for covering leftovers. They keep food fresh without any plastic, and you simply wash and reuse them.

SWAPS

Microwaving in plastic → Microwaving in glass
Zero leaching, no staining, lasts for decades.

Plastic lunchboxes → Stainless steel
Durable, safe, eco-friendly.

> ## Clingfilm → Beeswax wraps
> Reduce single-use plastics with a natural alternative.

At this point, you might be thinking: do I need to toss all my plastic containers and completely revamp my kitchen? Not necessarily. It's about priority and moderation. If you have a habit of microwaving food daily in plastic, that's a high-priority change — switch to glass for heating and you will have eliminated the main risk of plastic leaching. Hang on to your plastic tubs if you only use them for cold storage and never for hot.

I hope you don't feel all your kitchen equipment is out to poison you! My goal is not to sow fear, it is (always) to empower smarter choices. You're not going to keel over from using a Teflon pan or an occasional micro-waved plastic meal. However, we now know that small, consistent exposures to certain chemicals can add up over a lifetime. Making a few strategic swaps can dramatically reduce those exposures without throwing a wrench in your budget or convenience.

AND FINALLY...

That's it. The truth is, I'm just trying to share what I've learned to help others make better choices. This isn't a book about perfection or some ideal version of health. It's about what you can do today – starting with the choices you make when you shop. There's no magic three-month diet plan or eight-week ab programme here, just small, simple changes that add up over time. As Aubrey Marcus says, "Own the day, own your life." That's the point: get the little things right each day, and you'll find yourself living – and feeling – better.

And if Aubrey Marcus speaks to the everyday, Marcus Aurelius reminds us of the bigger picture: there are only three things worth caring about – your body, your purpose, and the people you share life with. Look after them, and you'll have all you need. Health is easy to take for granted until it's gone, but I hope this book helps you protect it – one shop, one meal, one choice at a time. Here's to your health, and thanks for reading.

ACKNOWLEDGEMENTS

This book wouldn't exist without my incredible wife, Anya. You've been my rock through every early morning, through every weekend working, every moment of doubt, and every bit of inspiration. Your unwavering belief in me, your patience when I disappeared into my work, and your constant love have carried me through this journey more than you'll ever know. To my sons, Jaxy and Bodhi, thank you for inspiring me every day to make the world a healthier place for your generation. And to the amazing team at Tonic Health, thank you for pushing our mission forward while I poured myself into this book. Your dedication makes everything possible. And finally, to everyone who's supported me along this journey, the community and those fighting every day to live a little healthier, thank you. This book is for you.

REFERENCES

INTRODUCTION

1   Jull, A. B., Cullum, N., Dumville, J. C., Westby, M. J., Deshpande, S., & Walker, N. (2015). Honey as a topical treatment for wounds. *Cochrane Database of Systematic Reviews*, 2015(3), CD005083. https://doi.org/10.1002/14651858. CD005083.pub4

2   Neri D., Steele E.M., Khandpur N., Cediel G., Zapata M.E., Rauber F., Marrón-Ponce J.A., Machado P., et al.; NOVA Multi-Country Study Group on Ultra-Processed Foods, Diet Quality and Human Health. Ultraprocessed food consumption and dietary nutrient profiles associated with obesity: A multicountry study of children and adolescents. *Obesity Reviews*, (23) Suppl 1:e13387. doi: 10.1111/obr.13387. Epub 2021 Dec 9. PMID: 34889015.

3   World Obesity Federation. (2024, March 4). *World Obesity Atlas 2024*. https://data.worldobesity.org/publications/WOF-Obesity-Atlas-v7.pdf

4   Office for Health Improvement and Disparities. (2025, May 7). *Obesity profile: Short statistical commentary, May 2025*. GOV. UK. https://www.gov.uk/government/statistics/obesity-profile-may-2025-update/obesity-profile-short-statistical-commentary-may-2025

5   UK Parliamentary Office of Science & Technology (POST). (2024, July 12). *Health impacts of ultra-processed foods (POSTbrief 0059)*. https://researchbriefings.files.parliament.uk/documents/POST-PB-0059/POST-PB-0059.pdf

6   https://researchbriefings.files.parliament.uk/documents/POST-PB-0059/POST-PB-0059.pdf

7   https://pubmed.ncbi.nlm.nih.gov/34889015/

8   Houshialsadat, Z., Cediel, G., & Machado, P. (2024). Ultra-processed foods, dietary diversity and micronutrient intakes in the Australian population. *European Journal of Nutrition*, 63(1), 135–144. https://doi.org/10.1007/s00394-023-03245-2

9   Chassaing, B., Koren, O., Goodrich, J. K., Poole, A. C., Srinivasan, S., Ley, R. E., & Gewirtz, A. T. (2015). Dietary emulsifiers impact the mouse gut microbiota promoting colitis

and metabolic syndrome. *Nature, 519*(7541), 92–96. https://
doi.org/10.1038/nature14232

10   Nigg, J. T., Lewis, K., Edinger, T., & Falk, M. (2012). Meta-
analysis of attention-deficit/hyperactivity disorder or attention-
deficit/hyperactivity disorder symptoms, restriction diet, and
synthetic food color additives. *Journal of the American Academy
of Child & Adolescent Psychiatry*, 51(1), 86–97.e8. https://doi.
org/10.1016/j.jaac.2011.10.015

11   International Agency for Research on Cancer. (2015, October
26). *IARC monographs evaluate consumption of red meat and
processed meat* (Press release No. 240). https://www.iarc.who.int/
wp-content/uploads/2018/07/pr240_E.pdf

12   Clear, J. (n.d.). "*Making a choice that is 1 percent better or 1
percent worse…*" JamesClear.com. https://jamesclear.com/
quotes/making-a-choice-that-is-1-percent-better-or-1-percent-
worse-seems-insignificant-in-the-moment-but-over-the-span-of-
moments-that-make-up-a-lifetime-these-choices-determine-the-
difference-betw

13   Brock, S. (2025, January 24). *5 ways to make healthy habits stick
– No willpower required.* Stanford Center on Longevity: Lifestyle
Medicine. https://longevity.stanford.edu/lifestyle/2025/01/24/
practice-of-the-month-create-and-maintain-your-new-healthy-
habit/

14   University College London. (2009, August 4). *How long does
it take to form a habit?* https://www.ucl.ac.uk/news/2009/aug/
how-long-does-it-take-form-habit

15   American Chemical Society. (2019, September 25). *Plastic
teabags release microscopic particles into tea. ScienceDaily.* https://
www.sciencedaily.com/releases/2019/09/190925083805.htm

FRUIT AND VEGETABLES

16   Ethnicity Facts and Figures. (2024, March 18). *Healthy eating
of 5 a day among adults.* GOV.UK. https://www.ethnicity-facts-
figures.service.gov.uk/health/diet-and-exercise/healthy-eating-of-
5-a-day-among-adults/latest/

17   Environmental Working Group (EWG). (2025). *EWG's 2025
Shopper's Guide to Pesticides in Produce™* – Full List. https://
www.ewg.org/foodnews/full-list.php

18   Office for Health Improvement and Disparities. (2024).
National Diet and Nutrition Survey (2019 to 2023) Report.
GOV.UK. https://www.gov.uk/government/statistics/national-

diet-and-nutrition-survey-2019-to-2023/national-diet-and-nutrition-survey-2019-to-2023-report

MILK

19 IBISWorld. (2025). *Liquid milk consumption per capita – United Kingdom industry report (44115)*. https://www.ibisworld.com/united-kingdom/bed/liquid-milk-consumption-per-capita/44115/

20 Ye, A., Singh, H., Taylor, M. W., & Anema, S. G. (2017). Interactions of milk proteins and fat globules during heat treatment and their influence on the structure of dairy products. *Journal of Dairy Science*, 100(5), 4151–4170. https://doi.org/10.3168/jds.2016-12094

21 Średnicka-Tober, D., Barański, M., Seal, C. J., Sanderson, R., Benbrook, C., Steinshamn, H., Gromadzka-Ostrowska, J., Rembiałkowska, E., Skwarło-Sońta, K., Eyre, M., Cozzi, G., Larsen, M. K., Jordon, T., Niggli, U., Sakowski, T., & Leifert, C. (2016). Composition differences between organic and conventional milk: A systematic literature review and meta-analysis. *British Journal of Nutrition*, 115(6), 1043–1060. https://doi.org/10.1017/S0007114516000349.

22 Tesco PLC. (2025). *Alpro Barista Coconut Long Life Dairy Free Drink*. https://www.tesco.com/groceries/en-GB/products/307741868

23 Sainsbury's. (2025). *Plenish Organic Almond Dairy-Free Drink 1L*. https://www.sainsburys.co.uk/gol-ui/product/plenish-organic-6-almond-dairy-free-drink-1l

Product references
https://www.tesco.com/groceries/en-GB/products/295790361
https://www.tesco.com/groceries/en-GB/products/275067782
https://www.sainsburys.co.uk/gol-ui/product/oatly-foamable-1l
https://www.sainsburys.co.uk/gol-ui/product/plenish-organic-6-almond-dairy-free-drink-1l

YOGHURT

24 The Guardian. (2023, April 6). *Yoghurt consumption trends in the UK: Health and dietary implications*. https://www.theguardian.com/business/2025/feb/01/full-fat-milk-sales-rise-uk-shoppers-leave-low-calorie-options

CHEESE

25 WorldAtlas. (2024). *Countries that consume the most cheese.* https://www.worldatlas.com/articles/countries-who-consume-the-most-cheese.html

26 Zhang, Y., Wang, M., Li, J., & Sun, Y. (2023). Associations of cheese consumption with cardiometabolic risk: A systematic review and meta-analysis. *Advances in Nutrition*, 14(6), 935–950. https://doi.org/10.1016/j.advnut.2023.08.001

EGGS

27 British Free Range Egg Producers Association (BFREPA). (2024). *Stocking density standards for free-range egg production.* https://www.bfrepa.co.uk/media-centre/stocking-density

28 Kühn, J., et al. (2014). Free-range farming: A natural alternative to produce vitamin D-enriched eggs. *World's Poultry Science Journal*, 70(4), 801–808. https://www.researchgate.net/publication/260556877_Free-range_farming_A_natural_alternative_to_produce_vitamin_D-enriched_eggs

Product references

Tesco PLC. (2025). *Tesco Free Range Eggs Medium 6 Pack.* https://www.tesco.com/groceries/en-GB/products/260298456

Tesco PLC. (2025). *Tesco Blueberries 150 g.* https://www.tesco.com/groceries/en-GB/products/287356888

Tesco PLC. (2025). *Bulk Greens Superfood Powder 100 g.* https://www.tesco.com/groceries/en-GB/products/315077398

Tesco PLC. (2025). *Fulfil Chocolate Salted Caramel Protein Bar 55 g* [Product page]. https://www.tesco.com/groceries/en-GB/products/315458345

MEAT AND FISH

29 Micha, R., Wallace, S. K., & Mozaffarian, D. (2010). Red and processed meat consumption and risk of incident coronary heart disease, stroke, and diabetes mellitus: A systematic review and meta-analysis. *Circulation*, 121(21), 2271–2283. https://doi.org/10.1161/circulationaha.109.924977

30 Wolk, A. (2017). Potential health hazards of eating red meat. *Journal of Internal Medicine*, 281(2), 106–122. https://doi.org/10.1111/joim.12543

31 Papier, K., Fensom, G. K., Knuppel, A., Appleby, P. N., Tong, T. Y. N., Schmidt, J. A., Travis, R. C., Key, T. J., & Perez-

Cornago, A. (2022). Meat consumption and risk of 25 common conditions: Outcome-wide analyses in 475,000 men and women in the UK Biobank study. *BMC Medicine*, 20(1), 240. https://pubmed.ncbi.nlm.nih.gov/33648505

32   Shakil MH, Trisha AT, Rahman M, Talukdar S, Kobun R, Huda N, Zzaman W. Nitrites in Cured Meats, Health Risk Issues, Alternatives to Nitrites: A Review. *Foods*. 2022 Oct 25;11(21):3355. doi: 10.3390/foods11213355. PMID: 36359973; PMCID: PMC9654915.

General references

Arnarson, A. (2024, April 18). Lean vs. fatty meat: Which is healthier? *Healthline*. https://www.healthline.com/nutrition/lean-vs-fatty-meat

WebMD. (2024). *Is grass-fed beef good for you?* Retrieved October 28, 2025, from https://www.webmd.com/diet/grass-fed-beef-good-for-you

Product references

Tesco PLC. (2025). *Tesco British Lean Beef Mince 5% Fat 500 g.* https://www.tesco.com/groceries/en-GB/products/300400644

Tesco PLC. (2025). *Tesco British Lean Beef Steak Minced.* https://www.tesco.com/groceries/en-GB/products/300400621

Tesco PLC. (2025). *Tesco British Chicken Breast Fillets.* https://www.tesco.com/groceries/en-GB/products/300400483

Tesco PLC. (2025). *Tesco Plant Chef Meat-Free Burgers.* https://www.tesco.com/groceries/en-GB/products/250871426

Tesco PLC. (2025). *Tesco Finest Sirloin Steak.* https://www.tesco.com/groceries/en-GB/products/308083458

Tonic Health. (2024, March 2). *Why choose grass-fed beef?* [Instagram reel]. Instagram. https://www.instagram.com/reel/C37sdW7IZSG/

PASTA, RICE AND GRAINS

33   Benton, D., Ruffin, M. P., Lassel, T., Nabb, S., Messaoudi, M., Vinoy, S., Desor, D., & Lang, V. (2007). The delivery rate of dietary carbohydrates affects cognitive performance in both rats and humans. *Psychopharmacology*, 192(3), 595–607. https://www.researchgate.net/publication/10984903_The_delivery_rate_of_dietary_carbohydrates_affects_cognitive_performance_in_both_rats_and_humans

Yours Magazine. (2024, September 9). *How much cereal should we be eating?* https://www.yours.co.uk/wellbeing/health/how-much-cereal-should-we-be-eating/

Product references

Tesco PLC. (2025). *Kellogg's Crunchy Nut Cereal 500g [Product page].* https://www.tesco.com/groceries/en-GB/products/256267349

Tesco PLC. (2025). *Kellogg's Coco Pops 480g.* Retrieved October 28, 2025, from https://www.tesco.com/groceries/en-GB/products/314605254

Tesco PLC. (2025). *Weetabix Cereal 24 Pack.* https://www.tesco.com/groceries/en-GB/products/254852996

Tesco PLC. (2025). *Nestlé Cheerios 390g.* https://www.tesco.com/groceries/en-GB/products/309177438

Tesco PLC. (2025). *Kellogg's Cornflakes 500g.* https://www.tesco.com/groceries/en-GB/products/303300896

Tesco PLC. (2025). *Kellogg's Frosties 500g.* Rhttps://www.tesco.com/groceries/en-GB/products/313748178

OILS

34 Newport MT, Dayrit FM. Analysis of 26 Studies of the Impact of Coconut Oil on Lipid Parameters: Beyond Total and LDL Cholesterol. *Nutrients.* 2025 Jan 30;17(3):514. doi: 10.3390/nu17030514. https://pmc.ncbi.nlm.nih.gov/articles/PMC11819987/4

BISCUITS

Product references

Tesco PLC. (2025). *McVitie's Rich Tea Biscuits 300 g.* https://www.tesco.com/groceries/en-GB/products/255404777

Tesco PLC. (2025). *Tesco Baked Cookies 200 g.* https://www.tesco.com/groceries/en-GB/products/283283133

Tesco PLC. (2025). *Fox's Chunkie Cookies 175 g.* https://www.tesco.com/groceries/en-GB/products/306650319

Tesco PLC. (2025). *McVitie's Chocolate Digestives 266 g.* https://www.tesco.com/groceries/en-GB/products/313008974

Tesco PLC. (2025). *McVitie's Digestives 400 g.* https://www.tesco.com/groceries/en-GB/products/313848238

Tesco PLC. (2025). *McVitie's Rich Tea Biscuits 300 g.* https://www.tesco.com/groceries/en-GB/products/255352138

Tesco PLC. (2025). *McVitie's Rich Tea Light Biscuits 300 g.* https://www.tesco.com/groceries/en-GB/products/255404777

CHOCOLATE AND SWEETS

Di Mattia, C. D., Martuscelli, M., Sacchetti, G., Beheydt, B., Mastrocola, D., & Pittia, P. (2011). Effect of cocoa processing on the antioxidant content of chocolate and cocoa powder. *BMC Chemistry*, 5(1), 5. https://doi.org/10.1186/1752-153X-5-5

Arnarson, A. (2023, May 12). 7 health benefits of dark chocolate. *Healthline.* https://www.healthline.com/nutrition/7-health-benefits-dark-chocolate

Product references

Tesco PLC. (2025). *Green Superfood Powder 100 g.* https://www.tesco.com/groceries/en-GB/products/317052482

Sainsbury's. (2025). *Naturya Organic Spirulina Powder 100 g* https://www.sainsburys.co.uk/gol-ui/product/naturya-spirulina--organic-100g

Tesco PLC. (2025). *Galaxy Smooth Milk Chocolate Bar 110 g* https://www.tesco.com/groceries/en-GB/products/314411984

Tesco PLC. (2025). *Tesco Dark Chocolate 200 g.* https://www.tesco.com/groceries/en-GB/products/260670257

Tesco PLC. (2025). *Lindt Excellence 70% Cocoa Dark Chocolate 100 g.* https://www.tesco.com/groceries/en-GB/products/259301725

Tesco PLC. (2025). *Lindt Excellence 85% Cocoa Dark Chocolate 100 g.* https://www.tesco.com/groceries/en-GB/products/250986325

Tesco PLC. (2025). *Lindt Excellence 90% Cocoa Dark Chocolate 100 g.* https://www.tesco.com/groceries/en-GB/products/264587407

Tesco PLC. (2025). *Maltesers Dark Chocolate Pouch 163 g.* https://www.tesco.com/groceries/en-GB/products/311947717

Tesco PLC. (2025). *M&M's Chocolate Pouch 125 g.* https://www.tesco.com/groceries/en-GB/products/303667679

Tesco PLC. (2025). *Galaxy Counters Chocolate Pouch 122 g.* https://www.tesco.com/groceries/en-GB/products/305832418

Tesco PLC. (2025). *Cadbury Dairy Milk Buttons 119 g.* https://www.tesco.com/groceries/en-GB/products/285383766

Tesco PLC. (2025). *Reese's Peanut Butter Cups 3-Pack.* https://www.tesco.com/groceries/en-GB/products/305963418

Tesco PLC. (2025). *Maltesers Milk Chocolate Pouch 135 g.* https://www.tesco.com/groceries/en-GB/products/305829106

SWEETS
Tesco PLC. (2025). *Haribo Fruitilicious Share Bag 160 g.* https://www.tesco.com/groceries/en-GB/products/308491637
Tesco PLC. (2025). *Haribo Starmix Share Bag 175 g.* https://www.tesco.com/groceries/en-GB/products/308482395
Tesco PLC. (2025). *Haribo Tangfastics Share Bag 175 g.* https://www.tesco.com/groceries/en-GB/products/308487211
Tesco PLC. (2025). *Haribo Supermix Share Bag 175 g.* https://www.tesco.com/groceries/en-GB/products/307740610
Tesco PLC. (2025). *Haribo Zingfest 175 g.* https://www.tesco.com/groceries/en-GB/products/310177719
Tesco PLC. (2025). *Rowntree's Berry Hearts 110 g.* https://www.tesco.com/groceries/en-GB/products/313623815
Tesco PLC. (2025). *Skittles Fruits Share Bag 152 g.* https://www.tesco.com/groceries/en-GB/products/314433923

COFFE AND TEA
Harvard T.H. Chan School of Public Health. (n.d.). *Coffee.* The Nutrition Source. https://nutritionsource.hsph.harvard.edu/food-features/coffee/.
Mayo Clinic Staff. (n.d.). *Caffeine: How much is too much?* Mayo Clinic. https://www.mayoclinic.org/healthy-lifestyle/nutrition-and-healthy-eating/in-depth/caffeine/art-20045678.
Nestlé Professional. (n.d.). *NESCAFÉ GOLD Cappuccino –* Ingredients. https://www.nestleprofessional.co.uk/coffee/nescafe-gold-cappuccino-1kg.
Plastic Pollution Coalition. (2022, July 15). *Make your coffee or tea plastic free.* https://www.plasticpollutioncoalition.org/blog/2022/07/15-plastic-free-coffee-tea.
National Center for Complementary and Integrative Health. (n.d.). *Tea and health.* https://www.nccih.nih.gov/health/tea.
Soil Association. (n.d.). *Why organic?* https://www.soilassociation.org/take-action/organic-living/why-organic/.
Hernandez, L. M., Yousefi, N., & Tufenkji, N. (2019). Plastic teabags release billions of microparticles and nanoparticles into tea. *Environmental Science & Technology*, 53(21), 12300–12310. https://doi.org/10.1021/acs.est.9b02540.

Banaei, G., et al. (2024). Teabag-derived micro/nanoplastics (true-to-life MNPLs) as a surrogate for real-life exposure scenarios. *Chemosphere*, 351, 143736. https://doi.org/10.1016/j.chemosphere.2024.143736.

SOFT DRINKS

35   Action on Sugar. (2018). *Survey: Confectionery sharing bags – sugar content and portion size.* https://www.actiononsugar.org/surveys/2018/confectionery-sharing-bags/

36   Hernandez, L. M., Yousefi, N., & Tufenkji, N. (2019). Plastic teabags release billions of microparticles and nanoparticles into tea. *Environmental Science & Technology*, 53(21), 12300–12310. https://doi.org/10.1021/acs.est.9b02540

37   Sylvetsky, A. C., & Rother, K. I. (2018). Trends in the consumption of low-calorie sweeteners: Advances in understanding their metabolic effects. *Frontiers in Nutrition*, 5, 68. https://pubmed.ncbi.nlm.nih.gov/27039282/

38   Consensus. (n.d.). *Are artificial sweeteners positive or negative for health?* https://consensus.app/search/are-artificial-sweeteners-positive-or-negative-for/i29HE2H6QOiBosJ0peYHHg/

ALCOHOL

39   GBD 2016 Alcohol Collaborators. (2018). Alcohol use and burden for 195 countries and territories, 1990–2016: A systematic analysis for the Global Burden of Disease Study 2016. *The Lancet*, 392(10152), 1015–1035. https://doi.org/10.1016/S0140-6736(18)30134-X

FREEZER SECTION

40   Carbon Brief. (2023, October 10). *Food waste makes up half of global food system emissions.* https://www.carbonbrief.org/food-waste-makes-up-half-of-global-food-system-emissions

Product references

Sainsbury's. (2025). *Blueberries (Frozen).* https://www.sainsburys.co.uk/gol-ui/SearchResults/blueberries

Sainsbury's. (2025). *Broccoli (Frozen).* https://www.sainsburys.co.uk/gol-ui/SearchResults/brocolli

Tesco PLC. (2025). *Spinach (Frozen).* https://www.tesco.com/groceries/en-GB/search?query=spinach

Tesco PLC. (2025). *Calippo Orange Ice Lolly 105 ml.* https://www.tesco.com/groceries/en-GB/products/313748633

Tesco PLC. (2025). *Twister Ice Lolly 80 ml.* https://www.tesco.com/groceries/en-GB/products/313376986

Tesco PLC. (2025). *Fab Strawberry Ice Lolly 58 ml.* https://www.tesco.com/groceries/en-GB/products/287129858

Tesco PLC. (2025). *Rowntree's Fruit Pastilles Lollies 4 Pack.* https://www.tesco.com/groceries/en-GB/products/254353778

Tesco PLC. (2025). *Del Monte Mango & Pineapple Lollies 3 Pack.* https://www.tesco.com/groceries/en-GB/products/263558565

Ocado. (2025). *Wall's Mini Milk Vanilla, Strawberry & Chocolate Ice Cream Lollies 12 Pack.* https://www.ocado.com/products/wall-s-mini-milk-vanilla-strawberry-chocolate-ice-cream-lollies-601974011

Ocado. (2025). *Little Jude's Milk Lollies 6 Pack.* https://www.ocado.com/products/little-jude-s-milk-lollies-392576011

Instagram. (2024, April 8). *Healthy swaps for frozen treats [Video].* https://www.instagram.com/tonichealth/reel/C7mF2X6ogQk/

KIDS' SWAPS

41   Agriculture and Horticulture Development Board (AHDB). (2023, September 4). *Ham and cheese sandwiches most popular back-to-school lunchbox items.* https://ahdb.org.uk/news/consumer-insight-ham-and-cheese-sandwiches-most-popular-back-to-school-lunchbox-items

42   World Health Organization (WHO) International Agency for Research on Cancer. (2015, October 26). *Cancer: Carcinogenicity of the consumption of red meat and processed meat.* https://www.who.int/news-room/questions-and-answers/item/cancer-carcinogenicity-of-the-consumption-of-red-meat-and-processed-meat

43   Imperial College London. (2023, February 13). *Ultra-processed foods make up almost two-thirds of Britain's diet, research shows.* https://www.imperial.ac.uk/news/238436/ultra-processed-foods-make-almost-two-thirds-britains/

44   BBC News. (2024, March 19). *Ultra-processed foods make up two-thirds of British diet, study finds.* https://www.bbc.co.uk/news/articles/cwy6g2dl44lo

PERSONAL CARE SWAPS

45   Choi, A. L., Sun, G., Zhang, Y., & Grandjean, P. (2012). Developmental fluoride neurotoxicity: A systematic review and meta-analysis. *Environmental Health Perspectives*, 120(10), 1362–1368. https://findresearcher.sdu.dk/ws/files/67397216/A237_ChoiEHPfluoride.pdf

46   Wang, L., Gao, H., Zhang, Y., & Liu, S. (2020). Cumulative risk assessment of paraben exposure from cosmetics. *Environment International*, 135, 105343. https://pubmed.ncbi.nlm.nih.gov/31903662/

47   Cancer Research UK. (2025). Sun safety and skin cancer prevention. https://www.cancerresearchuk.org/about-cancer/causes-of-cancer/sun-uv-and-cancer/sun-safety

48   The Skin Cancer Network. (2024). *European skin cancer news and prevention updates.* https://www.skincarenetwork.co.uk/skin-cancer-news/europe/

49   Journal of the American Academy of Dermatology. (2024). *Recent advances in understanding sunscreen safety.* https://www.sciencedirect.com/science/article/pii/S0022202X2400280X

50   Environmental Research. (2023). *Health impacts of cosmetic UV filters: A review.* https://www.sciencedirect.com/science/article/pii/S0160412023000120

51   European Commission, Scientific Committee on Consumer Safety (SCCS). (2021). *Opinion on ethylhexyl methoxycinnamate (EHMC)* (CAS No. 5466-77-3, EC No. 226-775-9). https://health.ec.europa.eu/publications/sccs-opinion-ethylhexyl-methoxycinnamate-ehmc-cas-no-5466-77-383834-59-7-ec-no-226-775-7629-661-9_en

52   Bentham Science Publishers. (2019). *Endocrine-disrupting effects of cosmetic ingredients: A comprehensive review.* https://www.eurekaselect.com/article/136872

53   Journal of Environmental and Public Health. (2023). *UV filters and human health risk assessment.* https://www.sciencedirect.com/science/article/abs/pii/S0946672X23001232

54   Alzheimer's Research UK. (2024). *Aluminium and Alzheimer's disease: Research update.* https://www.alzheimersresearchuk.org/news/aluminium-and-alzheimers/

55   International Academy of Oral Medicine and Toxicology (IAOMT). (n.d.). *Developmental fluoride neurotoxicity: Summary of Choi et al.* (2012). https://iaomt.org/choi-al-2012-

developmental-fluoride-neurotoxicity-systematic-review-meta-analysis/

56 National Toxicology Program (NTP). (2025). *Fluoride research and risk assessments.* https://ntp.niehs.nih.gov/research/assessments/noncancer/completed/fluoride

57 Meyer, F., Enax, J., Amaechi, B. T., Limeback, H., Fabritius, H. O., Ganss, B., Pawinska, M., & Paszynska, E. (2022). Hydroxyapatite as remineralization agent for children's dental care. *Frontiers in Dental Medicine*, 3, 859560. https://www.frontiersin.org/journals/dental-medicine/articles/10.3389/fdmed.2022.859560/full

General references
Toothpaste
NHS. (2023). *Fluoride.* https://www.nhs.uk/conditions/fluoride/

NHS England. (2022). *Hospital tooth extraction rates among children by local authority.* https://digital.nhs.uk/data-and-information/publications/statistical/hospital-dental-activity

Alzheimer's Research UK. (n.d.). *Aluminium and Alzheimer's disease.* https://www.alzheimersresearchuk.org/news/aluminium-and-alzheimers/

Cancer Research UK. (n.d.). *Deodorants and breast cancer risk.* https://www.cancerresearchuk.org/about-cancer/causes-of-cancer/cancer-myths-questions/cosmetics

European Food Safety Authority (EFSA). (2008). Safety of aluminium from dietary intake. *EFSA Journal*, 754, 1–34. https://doi.org/10.2903/j.efsa.2008.754

Scientific Committee on Consumer Safety (SCCS). (2018). Opinion on aluminium in cosmetic products (SCCS/1613/19). *European Commission.* hhttps://health.ec.europa.eu/document/download/c60cc5db-260d-4707-a75f-b994293a618b_en

Walker, V. R., et al. (2002). Antiperspirant use and the risk of breast cancer: A systematic review. *Journal of the National Cancer Institute*, 94(20), 1578–1580. https://doi.org/10.1093/jnci/94.20.1578

Parabens and cosmetics
Roberts, M. (2021). Parabens in cosmetics: An evidence review of risks and regulation. *Regulatory Toxicology and Pharmacology*, 125, 105005. https://doi.org/10.1016/j.yrtph.2021.105005

Schlumpf, M., Kypke, K., Wittassek, M., Angerer, J., Mascher, H., Mascher, D., & Lichtensteiger, W. (2008). Exposure patterns of parabens, phthalates, and benzophenone-3 in Swiss population samples: Comparison and implications. *International Journal of Hygiene and Environmental Health*, 211(5–6), 504–514. https://doi.org/10.1016/j.ijheh.2007.09.011

Scientific Committee on Consumer Safety (SCCS). (2011). Opinion on parabens (SCCS/1348/10). *European Commission*. https://ec.europa.eu/health/scientific_committees/consumer_safety/docs/sccs_o_041.pdf

Smith, K. W., Braun, J. M., Williams, P. L., Ehrlich, S., Correia, K. F., Calafat, A. M., Ye, X., Ford, J., Keller, M., Meeker, J. D., & Hauser, R. (2012). Predictors and variability of urinary paraben concentrations in men and women, including before and during pregnancy. *Environmental Health Perspectives*, 120(11), 1538–1543. https://pubmed.ncbi.nlm.nih.gov/22721761/

Matwiejczuk, N., Galicka, A., & Brzóska, M. M. (2020). Review of the safety of application of cosmetic products containing parabens. *Journal of Applied Toxicology*, 40(1), 176–210. https://doi.org/10.1002/jat.3917

Suncreams and UV filters

Cancer Research UK. (2025). *Sunscreen and sun safety*. https://www.cancerresearchuk.org/about-cancer/causes-of-cancer/sun-uv-and-cancer/sun-safety

Downs, C. A., Kramarsky-Winter, E., Segal, R., Fauth, J. E., Knutson, S., Bronstein, O., Ciner, F. R., Jeger, R., et al. (2021). Benzophenone accumulation from sunscreens and toxicity implications. *Chemical Research in Toxicology*, 34(3), 763–770. https://doi.org/10.1021/acs.chemrestox.0c00461

Krause, M., Klit, A., Blomberg Jensen, M., Søeborg, T., Frederiksen, H., Schlumpf, M., Lichtensteiger, W., Skakkebæk, N. E., & Drzewiecki, K. T. (2012). Sunscreens: Are they beneficial for health? An overview of endocrine-disrupting properties of UV filters. *International Journal of Andrology*, 35(3), 424–436. https://doi.org/10.1111/j.1365-2605.2012.01280.x

Schneider, S. L., & Lim, H. W. (2019). Review of environmental effects of oxybenzone and other sunscreen active ingredients. *Journal of the American Academy of Dermatology*, 80(1), 266–271. https://doi.org/10.1016/j.jaad.2018.06.033

Young, A. R., Narbutt, J., Harrison, G. I., Lawrence, K. P., Bell, M., & Wulf, H. C. (2021). Impact of sunscreen on vitamin D production: A systematic review. *British Journal of Dermatology*, 185(4), 733–741. https://doi.org/10.1111/bjd.20043

IARC. (2010). *Titanium dioxide. IARC Monographs on the Evaluation of Carcinogenic Risks to Humans*, 93.

U.S. Food and Drug Administration (FDA). (2022). *Sunscreen drug products for over-the-counter human use*. https://www.fda.gov

Chemical exposure and health risk context

National Toxicology Program (NTP). (2010). Toxicology and carcinogenesis studies of sodium lauryl sulfate in F344/N rats and B6C3F1 mice. https://ntp.niehs.nih.gov

National Cancer Institute (NCI). (2021). Antiperspirants/deodorants and breast cancer. https://www.cancer.gov/about-cancer/causes-prevention/risk/myths/antiperspirants-fact-sheet

Thomas, D., & Brusseau, M. (2014). Environmental transport and fate of chemicals (2nd ed.). Hoboken, NJ: John Wiley & Sons.

Office for National Statistics (ONS). (2023). Cancer registration statistics, England: 2022. https://www.ons.gov.uk

SUPPLEMENTS

58   Noah, L., Moreau, D., & Fardet, A. (2020). Changes in the mineral composition of foods: Evidence from 1940–2002. *Journal of Food Composition and Analysis*, 92, 103586. https://www.betterbiohealth.com/wp-content/uploads/2020/10/Mineral_Depletion_of_Foods_1940_2002.pdf

59   Young, L. M., Pipingas, A., White, D. J., Gauci, S., & Scholey, A. (2019). A systematic review and meta-analysis of B vitamin supplementation on depressive symptoms, anxiety, and stress: Effects on healthy and 'at-risk' individuals. *Nutrients*, 11(9), 2232. https://doi.org/10.3390/nu11092232

60   Linus Pauling Institute. (n.d.). *Micronutrient Inadequacies: the Remedy. Micronutrient Information Center*. Retrieved from https://lpi.oregonstate.edu/mic/micronutrient-inadequacies/remedy

61   NHS. (n.d.). *Vitamins for children – Weaning and feeding*. https://www.nhs.uk/baby/weaning-and-feeding/vitamins-for-children/#:~:text=Vitamin%20supplements,supplements%20at%20the%20same%20time.

62   Yang, Q., et al. (2025). Effectiveness of dietary supplements for skin photo-aging in healthy subjects: A review and meta-analysis

of 40 randomised controlled trials. *Frontiers in Medicine.* https://pubmed.ncbi.nlm.nih.gov/40761858/

63 Knaub, K., Schön, C., Alt, W., Durkee, S., Saiyed, Z., & Juturu, V. (2022). UC-II® undenatured type II collagen reduces knee joint discomfort and improves mobility in healthy subjects: A randomized, double-blind, placebo-controlled clinical study. *Journal of Clinical Trials,* 12, 492. https://www.longdom.org/open-access-pdfs/ucii-undenatured-type-ii-collagen-reduces-knee-joint-discomfort-and-improves-mobility-in-healthy-subjects-a-randomized-d.pdf

64 Pickering, G., Mazur, A., Trousselard, M., Bienkowski, P., Yaltsewa, N., Amessou, M., Noah, L., & Pouteau, E. (2020). Magnesium status and stress: The vicious circle concept revisited. *Nutrients,* 12(12), 3672. https://doi.org/10.3390/nu12123672

65 Oregon State University (2017). *Micronutrient Inadequacies in the US Population: an Overview.* https://lpi.oregonstate.edu/mic/micronutrient-inadequacies/overview

66 David Benton, Hayley A. Young, Do small differences in hydration status affect mood and mental performance?, *Nutrition Reviews,* Volume 73, Issue suppl_2, 1 September 2015, Pages 83–96, https://doi.org/10.1093/nutrit/nuv045

67 Adan, A. (2012). Cognitive performance and dehydration. *Journal of the American College of Nutrition,* 31(2), 71–78. https://www.researchgate.net/publication/230600141_Cognitive_Performance_and_Dehydration

CLEANING PRODUCTS

68 Arora, J., Ranjan, A., Chauhan, A., Biswas, R., et al. (2022). Surfactant pollution, an emerging threat to ecosystem: Approaches for effective bacterial degradation. *Journal of Applied Microbiology,* 133(3), 1229–1244. https://doi.org/10.1111/jam.15631

69 L'Oréal. MIT (Methylisothiazolinone) – Ingredient | Inside our products. https://inside-our-products.loreal.com/ingredients/mit

70 Rolsky, C. (2024, February 15). The controversy over PVA detergent pods. What it all means. *Shaw Institute.* https://shawinstitute.org/2024/02/15/the-controversy-over-pva-detergent-pods-what-it-all-means/

71 Rolsky, C., & Kelkar, V. (2021). Degradation of polyvinyl alcohol in US wastewater treatment plants and subsequent

nationwide emission estimate. *International Journal of Environmental Research and Public Health*, 18(11), 6027. https://doi.org/10.3390/ijerph18116027
72 de Groot, A. C. (2020). Fragrances: Contact allergy and other adverse effects. *Dermatitis*, 31(1), https://doi.org/10.1097/DER.0000000000000463

COOKING EQUIPMENT
73 Flinders University. (2022, October 31). *Not-so-tough Teflon.* https://news.flinders.edu.au/blog/2022/10/31/not-so-tough-teflon/
74 Plymouth Marine Laboratory. (2024, June 11). *New study shows plastic and non-stick cookware is likely adding thousands of microplastics into the human diet each year.* https://pml.ac.uk/news/new-study-shows-plastic-and-non-stick-cookware-is/
75 Liu, Y., et al. (2024). A systematic review of microplastics emissions in kitchens. *Environment International. Advance online publication.* https://doi.org/10.1016/j.envint.2024.108740
76 https://www.sciencedirect.com/science/article/pii/S016041202400326X
77 Stanford Medicine. (2025, January). *Microplastics and our health: What the science says.* https://med.stanford.edu/news/insights/2025/01/microplastics-in-body-polluted-tiny-plastic-fragments.html
78 Cancer-Research UK. (n.d.). *Does using plastic bottles and containers cause cancer?* https://www.cancerresearchuk.org/about-cancer/causes-of-cancer/cancer-myths-questions/does-using-plastic-bottles-and-containers-cause-cancer
79 Kumar, V., & Verma, P. (2025). Unveiling the hidden threat of micro-plastic in paper cups and tea bags: A critical review of their exacerbation and alarming concern in India. *Discover Applied Sciences*, 7(6), 1-32. https://doi.org/10.1007/s42452-025-07121-y

General references
Bergmann, M. et al. (2019) 'Plastic pollution in the global ocean: an overview of the current state and future challenges', *Nature Reviews Earth & Environment*, 1, pp. 47–60. doi:10.1038/s43017-019-0001-3.
News Desk (2022) *Notsotough Teflon. Flinders University News*, published 31 October. Available at: https://news.flinders.edu.au/blog/2022/10/31/not-so-tough-teflon/

Plymouth Marine Laboratory, 2024. *New study shows plastic and nonstick cookware is likely adding thousands of microplastics into the human diet.* [online] Plymouth Marine Laboratory. Available at: https://pml.ac.uk/news/new-study-shows-plastic-and-non-stick-cookware-is/ [Accessed 1 August 2025].

Liu, M., Brandsma, S. H. & Schreder, E., 2024. *From ewaste to living space: Flame retardants contaminating household items add to concern about plastic recycling. Chemosphere*, 365, p. 143319. Corrigendum published in *Chemosphere*, 370, p. 143903 (2025).

Zhang, Y. et al. (2024) 'A systematic review of microplastics emissions in kitchens', *Environment International*, 187, p. 109770.

Birnbaum, L.S. and Cohen Hubal, E.A. (2006) 'Polyfluoroalkyl chemicals: an emerging threat to public health?', *Environmental Health Perspectives*, 114(5), pp. 313–315. doi:10.1289/ehp.114-a313.

Cancer Research UK (2023) *Plastic food packaging and cancer risk.* [online] Available at: https://www.cancerresearchuk.org/about-cancer/causes-of-cancer/cancer-controversies/plastics [Accessed 30 Jul 2025].

Chen, Q. et al. (2020) 'Microplastics in food: health risks and food chain contamination', *Journal of Agricultural and Food Chemistry*, 68(17), pp. 4833–4845. doi:10.1021/acs.jafc.0c00120.

European Chemicals Agency (ECHA) (2023) *Proposal to restrict PFAS.* [online] Available at: https://echa.europa.eu/restrictions-under-consideration/-/substance-rev/72301/term [Accessed 30 Jul 2025].

Environment Agency (UK) (2022) *Forever chemicals: review of PFAS pollution.* [online] Available at: https://researchbriefings.files.parliament.uk/documents/POST-PN-0747/POST-PN-0747.pdf

Gao, X. et al. (2021) 'Release of microplastics from polypropylene containers under simulated microwave heating', *Science of the Total Environment*, 763, 144247. doi:10.1016/j.scitotenv.2020.144247.

Greenpeace UK (2023) *Toxic utensils: hidden hazards in black plastic kitchenware.* [online] Available at: https://share.upmc.com/2025/03/black-plastic-cookware/#:~:text=Why%20Did%20the%20Study%20Cause,releasing%20harmful%20substances%20into%20food

Health and Safety Executive (HSE) (2024) *Decabromodiphenyl ether (decaBDE) – UK restriction.* [online] https://www.gov.uk/government/publications/brominated-flame-retardants-properties-incident-management-and-toxicology/brominated-flame-retardants-decabromodiphenyl-ether-general-information

IKEA UK (2024) *IKEA 365+ food containers product safety information.* [online] Available at: https://www.ikea.com/gb/en/p/ikea-365-food-container-glass [Accessed 30 Jul 2025].

Kwiatkowski, C.F. et al. (2020) 'Scientific basis for managing PFAS as a chemical class', *Environmental Science & Technology Letters*, 7(8), pp. 532–543. doi:10.1021/acs.estlett.0c00255.

National Institute for Health and Care Excellence (NICE) (2021) *Environmental toxicology guidance for consumer products.* https://www.nice.org.uk/guidance/ng70

Parliamentary Environmental Audit Committee (UK) (2025) *PFAS: 'Forever Chemicals' in the Environment Inquiry.* [online] Available at: https://committees.parliament.uk/work/7289/pfas-forever-chemicals-in-the-environment [Accessed 30 Jul 2025].

Rochman, C.M. et al. (2015) 'Policy: Classify plastic waste as hazardous', *Nature*, 494, pp. 169–171. doi:10.1038/494169a.

Rogers, B.P. et al. (2022) 'Exposure to microplastics through culinary utensils: risk analysis', *Food and Chemical Toxicology*, 161, 112844. doi:10.1016/j.fct.2022.112844.

Rosenmai, A.K. et al. (2014) 'Are structural analogues to bisphenol A safe alternatives?', *Toxicological Sciences*, 139(1), pp. 35–47. doi:10.1093/toxsci/kfu030.

Tefal UK (2023) *PFAS-free cookware and product safety certifications.* [online] Available at: https://blog.tefal.co.uk/2024/04/16/the-non-stick-material-ptfe-of-tefal-pans-everything-you-need-to-know/

UK Government (2024) *Single-use plastics ban comes into force.* [online]. Available at: https://www.gov.uk/government/news/new-bans-and-restrictions-on-polluting-single-use-plastics-come-into-force

US National Toxicology Program (2016) *Toxicology studies of perfluorooctanoic acid (PFOA).* [online] Available at: https://ntp.niehs.nih.gov/research/assessments/noncancer/completed/pfoa

Wang, Z. et al. (2017) 'A never-ending story of per- and polyfluoroalkyl substances (PFASs)?', *Environmental Science & Technology*, 51(5), pp. 2508–2518. doi:10.1021/acs.est.6b04806.

INDEX

ABOUT THE AUTHOR

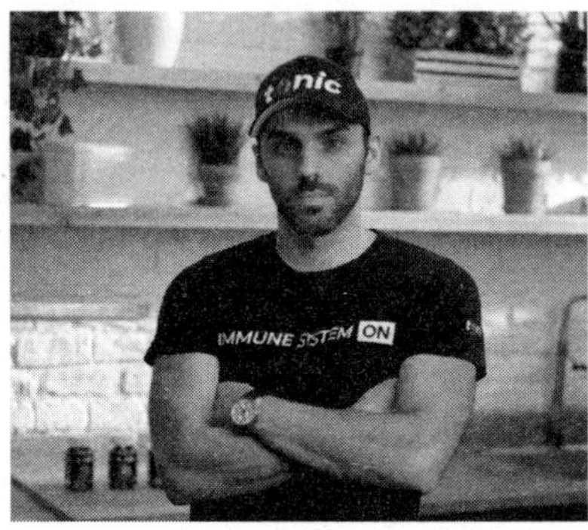

Sunna van Kampen is the founder of
Tonic Health, which aims to tackle the UK's
nutrient deficiency crisis by providing nutrition
advice for real life. Tonic is now the UK's fastest-
growing vitamin brand and stocked in over 10,000+
distribution points including every major
retailer in the UK. He lives in Devon with
his wife and two children.